Narrative Systems in Psychotherapy

Narrative Systems in Psychotherapy

AN INTEGRATIVE APPROACH TO INDIVIDUAL,
COUPLE, AND FAMILY THERAPY

FIRST EDITION

Geoffrey Buckley, Ph.D.

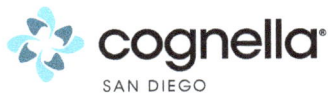

cognella®

SAN DIEGO

Bassim Hamadeh, CEO and Publisher
Amy Smith, Project Editor
Emely Villavencio, Senior Graphic Designer
Stephanie Kohl, Licensing Coordinator
Natalie Piccotti, Director of Marketing
Kassie Graves, Vice President of Editorial
Jamie Giganti, Director of Academic Publishing

cognella® | ACADEMIC PUBLISHING
3970 Sorrento Valley Blvd., Ste. 500, San Diego, CA 92121

BRIEF CONTENTS

Preface xiii

CHAPTER 1   Introduction to Narrative Systems
Theory   1

CHAPTER 2   The Story Within   7

CHAPTER 3   Healing, Holding, Helping   15

CHAPTER 4   Love Stories   23

CHAPTER 5   Stories of Temperament, Attraction, and
Negotiating Perceptions   29

CHAPTER 6   The Story of Emotion,
Part 1: *Understanding*   37

CHAPTER 7   The Story of Emotion,
Part 2: *Expressing*   49

CHAPTER 8   The Story of Communication   55

CHAPTER 9   The Story of Relationships   65

CHAPTER 10   The Story of Healthy Marriages   75

CHAPTER 11   The Story of Conflict   81

CHAPTER 12   The Story About Helping Couples   87

CHAPTER 13   Family Stories   105

CHAPTER 14   Matching Your Therapeutic Approach to the
Family   113

CHAPTER 15   Thoughts on Therapy and Culture   119

Appendix   125
Index   147

DETAILED CONTENTS

Preface   xiii

CHAPTER 1

Introduction to Narrative Systems Theory   1

Chapter Summary and Learning Objective   1
Questions for Discussion   6

CHAPTER 2

The Story Within   7

Chapter Summary and Learning Objective   7
Questions for Discussion   13

CHAPTER 3

Healing, Holding, Helping   15

Chapter Summary and Learning Objective   15
Healing   15
Holding   17
Helping   19
Questions for Discussion   21

CHAPTER 4

Love Stories   23

Chapter Summary and Learning Objective   23
Attraction and Attachment   23
Attachment Styles   25
Questions for Discussion   27

CHAPTER 5

Stories of Temperament, Attraction, and Negotiating Perceptions   29

Chapter Summary and Learning Objective   29
Temperament   29
Reenactment   30
Memory   31
Choices   32
Negotiating Perceptions   33
Truth and Motive   34
Questions for Discussion   36

CHAPTER 6

The Story of Emotion, Part 1: *Understanding*   37

Chapter Summary and Learning Objective   37
Primary Emotions   37
The Color of Emotion   39
Secondary Emotions   43
Angst   46
Questions for Discussion   48

CHAPTER 7

The Story of Emotion, Part 2: *Expressing*   49

Chapter Summary and Learning Objective   49
Emotional Honesty   49
Questions for Discussion   53

CHAPTER 8

The Story of Communication   55

Chapter Summary and Learning Objective   55
Confusing Messages   55

Dealing with Defenses   58
The Parent, Adult, Child Model   60
    Parent   60
    Child   61
    Adult   61
Questions for Discussion   63

CHAPTER 9

The Story of Relationships   65

Chapter Summary and Learning Objective   65
A Counseling Session   65
Content and Process   67
Personalities   72
Problems   72
Questions for Discussion   73

CHAPTER 10

The Story of Healthy Marriages   75

Chapter Summary and Learning Objective   75
A Healthy Marriage   75
Valuing   76
Belonging   76
Enjoying   77
Practicing Playfulness   77
Deals, Feelings, and Fun   79
Making Deals   79
Questions for Discussion   80

CHAPTER 11

The Story of Conflict   81

Chapter Summary and Learning Objective   81
The Purpose of Conflict   81
Questions for Discussion   85

CHAPTER 12

The Story About Helping Couples   87

Chapter Summary and Learning Objective   87
Your Treatment Plan   87
Approaches to Therapy   88
Thoughts, Feelings, Behaviors   89
Insight-Oriented Therapies   89
Behavior-Oriented Therapies   90
Emotionally Focused Therapy   90
Where Do We Start?—Where Are We Headed?   91
Principles of Change   93
Your Next Session   96
   Strategy 1: Develop a Clear Understanding of Each Partner's Contribution to Problems in the Relationship, Exposing the "Circular Causality" That Reinforces Ongoing Conflicts.   97
   Strategy 2: Create Guidelines and Agreements for Containing Hurtful and Defensive Behaviors.   97
   Strategy 3: Access and Clarify Emotionally Charged Issues and Behaviors; Encourage Vulnerability, Empathy, and Mutual Caring.   97
   Strategy 4: Develop Guidelines and Strategies for Constructive Conflict and Effective Communication.   98
   Strategy 5: Emphasize the Couple's Strengths and Encourage Positive, Caring Behaviors.   98
   Applying Christensen's Strategies   98
Questions for Discussion   104

CHAPTER 13

Family Stories   105

Chapter Summary and Learning Objective   105
Families Defined   106
Family Dynamics   106
Family Stressors   107
Family Systems   107
Family Differentiation, Motivation, and Openness to Change   108
Family Therapy, Eight Approaches   109
   Experiential Family Therapy   109
   Narrative Family Therapy   109

Psychodynamic and Transgenerational Family Therapy   109
Cognitive-Behavioral Family Therapy   110
Structural Family Therapy   110
Strategic Family Therapy   110
Solution-Focused Family Therapy   110
An Integrative Approach   110
Questions for Discussion   111

CHAPTER 14

Matching Your Therapeutic Approach to the Family   113

Chapter Summary and Learning Objective   113
Finding the Best Approach to Treating Your Client Family   113
Questions for Discussion and Exercises   116
Exercise #1: Differentiation   116
Exercise #2: Family Rules   117
Exercise #3: Family Roles   117
Exercise #4: Family Rituals   117
Exercise #5: Genogram   118

CHAPTER 15

Thoughts on Therapy and Culture   119

Chapter Summary and Learning Objective   119
Listening with Your Head, Heart, and Spirit   120
On the Sacredness of Therapy   120
Questions for Discussion   122
Becoming an Effective Multicultural Counselor   122
Beliefs and Attitudes   122
Knowledge   122
Skills and Intervention Strategies   123

Appendix   125

Effective Communication   125
Speaking and Listening   125
Guidelines for Effective Communication   126

1. Use Discretion and Good Timing   126

2. Take Turns   127

3. Talk About Yourself, Your Own Feelings   127

4. Stay in the "Here and Now"   128

5. Give Feedback   129

From Lecture to Lab   131

6. Use "Time-Outs"   131

7. Have a "Postmortem"   132

Preparing for the Postmortem   133

The Archeology of Relationship   134

Guidelines for Good Communication Handout   135

Guidelines for Good Communication Handout   135

Discussion Questions About Emotions   136

Discussion Questions About Defenses   136

Discussion Questions About Messages   137

Common "Feeling Words"   137

Modified Differentiation of Self Scale   138

Parenting Plan   140

Marriage Survey   142

Index   147

PREFACE

've been working on this book for the past 30 years. I'm a slow writer. One reason that it's taken so long is that I haven't been sure who my audience was. I first wrote a workbook for couples—something I could give clients to help them understand and more actively participate in couples therapy. In the workbook I included chapters about the typical types of conflicts that couples deal with, how emotions and defenses can get in the way, and how to develop strategies for managing emotions, resolving conflicts, and becoming better friends. I also included exercises for couples to do between sessions in order to practice skills and enhance feelings of closeness and intimacy.

The workbook was done, but a few years ago I got the bright idea to write a sourcebook for my students in the couple counseling classes I teach in graduate schools. I wanted to research some of the most effective approaches currently used by other clinicians to determine which approaches I could recommend to my students. In the process, I discovered some of the most recent methods of integrating counseling theories with clinical practice and became fascinated with the possibility of helping students recognize the typical problems and patterns that couples struggle with and the best ways to help them.

Before long I realized I was having too much fun with the reading and research and needed to get back to writing. So I decided to put these two books together into one. My idea was to write a workbook for clients that could also benefit students and even practicing therapists who wanted to refresh their skills. It wasn't a good idea. It's too difficult to do both—to create a sourcebook for students interested in the academics of counseling theories that could also hold the interest of couples in therapy. I had originally planned to go behind the curtain to let clients and students into my thoughts about why I make the choices I make when I'm working with couples. Because I like teaching, I often find myself wanting to let clients in on what's going on with their therapy, why we're doing what we're doing, and why I think it will help. I still think that may be interesting to some clients, but I've decided to rewrite the couple therapy workbook to make it less academic and easier to use.

This book is for students. It could be called a sourcebook because I plan to introduce a variety of therapeutic approaches that work with couples and families. I also plan to introduce many of the books I recommend to both students and couples. I'll comment on the approaches I think work best with different client populations. I included an appendix with exercises that I give to couples for homework. Feel free to use any of the handouts or exercises.

Malcolm Gladwell said that it takes 10,000 hours of practice to become an expert at something.[1] I've been a marriage counselor for over 35 years, working with 15 to 20 couples a week, 48 weeks a year. The math isn't difficult. And I'm happy to say that the majority of those couples report doing much better. Most of what I will be

---

1 Gladwell, M. (2008). *Outliers.*

sharing with you in this book has been said by others. That's very good news. It's good news when many professionals, looking at what works and doesn't work in relationships, report similar findings and offer similar advice. So my plan is to synthesize, emphasize, and illustrate what works best in counseling with individuals, marriages, and families. I will be reviewing some of the latest research and offering my own experiences as well as case studies to help you quickly target common problem areas and develop the skills and insight you need to help your clients resolve the most common types of conflicts.

There already exist very good books on marriage and relationships. I will be reviewing many of them in the pages that follow. The problem is that so many books on marriage rely too heavily on good ideas and information. Ideas and information are certainly important, but the emphasis in this book will be helping your client couples learn to develop skills. That's why I plan to distill and summarize the most important lessons I've learned from working with couples over the years and emphasize the skills and strategies that work.

As I've said, information about why problems occur in relationships, and ideas about how to fix them, are certainly useful and important. It's good to have insight into oneself and one's partner. It's good to have insight into various conflict patterns and trigger issues. Insight and understanding are important for acceptance, and acceptance is fundamental to trust and the ability to find solutions. But understanding alone won't do the job. If it did, self-help books would be much more effective. We wouldn't need coaches, piano teachers, AA sponsors, or golf pros. Marriage therapists, who should know better, frequently rely too heavily on providing insight. Insight is less useful than most people think; with luck, it may be 20 percent of what helps people change. To get along with each other, talk through problems, and negotiate solutions, couples need to learn and practice skills. Learning skills involves effort, but I can think of no more important skills to practice than the skills needed to have a successful and loving relationship.

Acknowledgments

I would like to thank my wife, Kathleen, and my three daughters, Bethany, Amee, and Elizabeth, for their support, encouragement, and help in the development of this book.

I would also like to thank my professors and colleagues for their instruction and inspiration, especially Ray Anderson, Ph.D., of Fuller Theological Seminary; Mary Margaret Thomas, Ph.D., of California Lutheran University; Dennis Patrick Slattery, Ph.D., of Pacifica Graduate Institute; Rie Rogers Mitchell, Ph.D., of California State University Northridge; and Barbara Ingram, Ph.D., of Pepperdine University.

CHAPTER ONE

Introduction to Narrative Systems Theory

We live inside of stories

CHAPTER SUMMARY AND LEARNING OBJECTIVE

Chapter 1 introduces the idea that the brain habitually creates an internal narrative in order to organize and make sense of experience. Because the brain is a story teller, all approaches to psychotherapy can be understood as narrative systems—a storyline which adds structure to thought. While established psychotherapeutic approaches can be thought to be valid and useful in themselves, each approach is a form of language, a story about people and how to help people with mental and emotional problems. This chapter emphasizes the importance of thoroughly understanding each theoretical orientation, that is, how, and in what contexts, each theoretical approach works best. In this way, one or more therapeutic approaches can be effectively tailored to the client's problem. When the clinician can conceptualize each therapeutic approach as a language system it is easier to detect the commonalities of each approach and effectively integrate elements of treatment.

The learning objective for this chapter is to familiarize students with a completely novel method of understanding and applying theoretical approaches to clinical treatment.

Therapists listen to stories—many stories, day after day and week after week. We listen to stories about pain and heartache, about betrayal and trauma, about confusion, frustration, and exhaustion. Our training provides us with many ways of listening to our client's story and many ways to respond. It's important to know whether the story we are listening to is our client's story or our own.

We live inside the stories that our brains tell in order to make sense of ourselves, our experiences, and the world around us. Dan Siegel tells us that our brains narrativize experience and self-awareness, creating autobiographical memory. The resulting *schema* informs our perceptions, beliefs, automatic thoughts, and the emotional imprinting from which we construct our reality. As you listen to your client tell his or her story in therapy, you'll notice how the story reaches into the past for illustrations, circles around present problems, and anticipates the challenges of the future. You will have to construct this format yourself, however, since stories told in therapy rarely follow a linear progression. Your client's brain searches for antecedents and consequences with which to create a narrative—an accumulation and re-presentation of events and meaning selected to invite you into his or her inner life and the challenges your client faces. What story are you listening to? What is the story your brain is telling you about the story your client is telling? The purpose of this chapter is to help you to answer that question—to help you become more conscious of the many story options you have with which to better *hear* the story you are listening to.

The theoretical orientations you study in your training to become a psychotherapist provide a library of storied possibilities. You study "psychodynamic" stories about people as they grow and develop, about their early attachments and object relations, about their family and cultural conditioning, their developmental milestones, and the impact of childhood wounds. These are stories about how the effects of the past continue to inform and challenge the story we are living today. You study "cognitive" and "behavioral" stories about how thoughts, feelings, and behaviors are all interrelated, and that each domain is impacted by the choices we make and rehearse. Your training enables you to become more conscious of the central task of therapy—to enable your clients to become more aware of the choices they have inside of their own stories. You will help them realize that perception itself is a choice—that they have options in choosing how they think, feel, and behave. And the goal of your work will be to help your clients become more skillful in making healthier and more adaptive choices.

Freedom, choice, and response-ability are terms you become familiar with as you learn about the "existential" story of human experience. Many of your clients will be trying to make sense of their lives and to find meaning in the problems they face. Others of your clients are trying to make better choices in their relationships, set better boundaries, and deal more successfully with their families. In family therapy, you will help them to be aware of the impact of their families of origin and to be more conscious of healthy ways to think, feel, and behave more independently, as separate and unique individuals with the ability to respond from the choice to love rather than to react from guilt or shame.

The families we grow up in, the cultural norms and expectations surrounding us, and our life experiences create our stories. We cannot abstract ourselves from the influence of the story we live in or the language in which we experience that story. Language lifts experience into consciousness. Language enlivens and deepens experience into story. The diverse studies in the multifaceted languages of your profession equip you to listen more deeply into the stories you are being told in therapy and to hear those stories against the background of the many psychological languages you have been taught. Your colleagues (Freud, Klein, Skinner, Rogers, Ainsworth, Fromm, and many others) each contribute a unique experience and vantage point—each telling his or her own story about human nature. Some stories may be more interesting or seem more relevant but, together, they are an essential collection of narratives that reveal truths about the human story.

As you listen to each of these story tellers, you soon begin to see overlapping motifs, common perspectives, and therapeutic approaches. The systemic relatedness of individual psychological narratives combine to enrich your perspectives of human nature and human difficulties. Listening to your clients tell you about their struggles, their challenges, and the stories they choose to illustrate these challenges will reveal not only their problems but also the way in which they perceive their problems. The host of theoretical orientations you study becomes the narrative genre that informs your choices of what to hear and how to respond. You and your client work within a systemic matrix to develop and expand upon a shared therapeutic narrative. In *The Neuroscience of Psychotherapy* (2002), Louis Cozolino affirms that

> Interpretations in psychodynamic therapy, exposure in behavioral thera- pies, or experiments in differentiation from a family systems perspective all focus on this goal. Through the activation of multiple cognitive and emotional networks, previously dissociated functions are integrated and gradually brought under the control of cortical executive functions. Narratives co-constructed with therapists provide a new template for thoughts, behaviors, and ongoing integration.[1]

The brain is a story teller. It organizes and interprets experience influenced by myriad associations of past and ongoing experience. The interconnected systems of life and language create narratives of meaning. What kind of story is being told? Patient and therapist work together to listen *into* the story, to discover the how and why of the story, to find the meaning and means to positively move the story forward.

Therapy is well described as the talking cure. The talking cure is a quest to create a better story, a healthier, healing story. It is the therapist's quest as much as the patient's. "We are kept there (in the therapeutic process) by the sense of wanting something deeply important."[2] That something has been referred to as an "aesthetic imperative"; it is the gripping immediacy of emerging motifs come to life in the patient's story. The therapist, tutored in the psyche's various languages, will hear those motifs repeated not only in psychological genre but in the voice of film, art, and literature as well.

> The therapist is aware of the aesthetic imperative (of these literary motifs) as he listens to what the patient says, and feels, its affective thrust. ... The reason for this profound vitality which all sense in the words of men like Dante, Goethe, or Shakespeare is simply that they traffic continually in archetypal symbols and emotions.[3]

The stories told in therapy are told in order to bridge the space between—the space in which therapist and patient work closely together to *right* the patient's story. What happens to the teller and to the listener in that space? Both are transformed in the systemic narrative that presents itself among the countless possibilities of shared language and experience and opens to that aesthetic imper- ative of mutual discovery. And because language is systemic, spoken and heard from storied contexts, your professional training equips you to think in the larger context of a multitude of possible ways in which to hear and respond to your patient's story.

Your professional training equips you with languages of your profession. But more than providing you with a vast vocabulary of terms and concepts, you learn to recognize which languages and stories work best in which contexts. I discuss

---

1   Cozolino, L. (2002). *The Neuroscience of Psychotherapy*, p. 170.
2   Hillman, J. (1975). *Revisioning Psychology.*
3   Cox M., & Theilgaard, A. (1987). *Mutative Metaphors in Psychotherapy*, p. 31.

four contexts in this book: stories that describe individuals, stories that describe relationships, stories that describe families, and stories that describe the impact of culture. These stories are all related. They must be. There cannot be a story about a relationship apart from the story of the individuals in the relationship or the families and culture in which those individuals have been birthed. The days of clinicians stubbornly clinging to a single theoretical orientation about human experience are past. People are too dynamic and complex. It's best to think of theoretical orientations as useful and interesting stories and to be well versed in the *whys* and *ways* to apply each story.

Most therapists today tend to develop an integrative approach to therapy that incorporates important aspects of various theoretical perspectives depending on the presenting problem. They have learned to speak systemic languages in order to listen more deeply to their patient's story, to discover the multifaceted dynamics of the story, and to find the meaning and means to select the best stories with which to understand and respond to their patient's story. A simplistic illustration of the relatedness of psychological languages is to imagine a compass rose. A ship's helmsman steers a course guided by the ship's compass. The therapist steers the course of therapy guided by an internal compass—the ability to match the treatment direction and plan to the presenting problem(s) of the client. Clearly the ability to steer the right course depends on his or her ability to navigate the many potential directions a course of treatment may require. A therapist's skill as a navigator is tested by the strong and varied currents of conversations present in a typical hour of therapy.

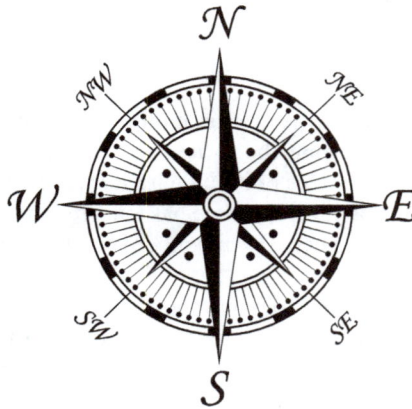

FIG. 1-1
Copyright © 2014 Depositphotos/Seamartini.

While there are four main points of the mariner's compass: north, south, east, and west, the therapist's compass must include a fifth point. The five main compass directions that occur in psychotherapy are psychodynamic, humanistic/existential, cognitive-behavioral, systemic, and medical/biological.

The psychodynamic direction is about "what happened." What happened in a person's life that has contributed to his or her development? What attachment issues or object relations were at work in a person's early life? What were the dynamics of social and familial conditioning? What types of life experiences or traumas might have occurred?

A psychodynamic perspective provides not only insight into these issues but also an opportunity to work through or heal much of these developmental conflicts. The humanistic/existential direction is about "what's important." The work of Carl Rogers and Abraham Maslow were foundational in what has been called the humanistic or human potential movement. Roger's was confident that when a therapist offers unconditional positive regard, empathic warmth, and genuineness, the client will be able to overcome the all-too-common "conditions of worth" that limit human potential. That potential is fully realized when one has managed to meet basic survival needs, has experienced belongness and love, and has reached a quality of self-esteem that opens to the possibility of self-actualization—the confluence of *doing* with *being*. This striving to be an authentic *Self*, facing life and death courageously and embracing the freedom that comes with the response-ability of being fully alive, describes the existential goal of creating meaning and striving for what is truly important in life.

Changing one's behavior and ways of thinking requires practice. The cognitive -behavioral direction on the clinician's therapeutic compass is "what's needed." What everyone needs is to acquire the insights and behaviors essential for mature living. A mature individual examines his or her thoughts and beliefs in the light of reality and sober, healthy decision-making. Mature decisions are made in spite of, or in the face of, difficult emotions. Growth in maturity requires learning and rehearsing these skills.

It's been said that culture is the sea we swim in. We are continually influenced by family, cultural, and philosophical systems. Consequently, one's therapeutic compass must also point in a systemic direction. A systems perspective helps us to understand "what's involved" in the process of navigating the complex and multifaceted nature of being human. No current textbook in the field of clinical training fails to review the important steps to becoming culturally sensitive. It's also essential to have a thorough understanding of how families influence thoughts, beliefs, and behavior. The rules, roles, and rituals that we grow up with condition our world view, values, and perceptions. Because of this, each new client we interview, regardless of apparent similarities, represents a cross-cultural encounter requiring curiosity and genuine respect for different family experiences.

The fifth direction in therapy is the need to consider physical and biological issues. Issues such as sleep problems, chronic pain, physical injury, and other health-related problems certainly influence the process and outcome of therapy. The most common concern for therapists may be the need to refer a client to a physician for medication. Serious problems with depression, anxiety, sleep disorders, and many other types of psychological disorders should not be treated with talk therapy alone.

A skilled clinician speaks many psychological languages. People present with a variety of problems that call for a variety of theoretical perspectives and approaches. It's good when a therapist can quickly and intuitively grasp the best direction and intervention to use with a patient. Sometimes the focus will be on present problems, sometimes on past effects. The focus may be on disruptive thoughts, feelings, or behaviors. Whatever the focus, that intuitive approach must arise from a solid foundation of clinical training. To that end, I agree with the authors of *A General Theory of Love*:

Strip away a therapist's orientation, the books on his shelves, the meetings he attends—the cognitive framework his rational mind demands—and what is left to define the psychotherapy he conducts? Himself ... The dispensable trappings of dogma may determine what a therapist thinks he is doing, what he talks about when he talks about therapy, but the agent of change is who he is.[4]

One finds the affirmation above repeated frequently in psychological literature. Current textbooks on counseling techniques, individual, couple, and family therapies all agree that *you*, the therapist, are the catalyst of change. Carl Rogers, with his research into the healing properties of psychotherapy, was possibly the most articulate on this point. But while I agree with the quote, I'm fairly sure that the authors take for granted that the agent of change, the therapist, has thoroughly learned his or her craft. An accomplished artist has mastered technique so thoroughly that the brush seems to be directing itself. My artist friend is often asked the question, "how long did it take to paint this?" He enjoys answering, "40 years."

Just so, a competent therapist has skillfully and intelligently integrated and refined his or her theoretical insights. And those insights find their common roots in the fundamental truths and stories about what people feel and need. He or she may prefer a specific theoretical approach, but, ideally, that approach has been carefully selected from a clear understanding of its advantages and disadvantages relative to other approaches and against the backdrop of the therapist's own unique personality style and clinical strengths.

We live inside of stories. This text adds yet another story. I will be talking about the interrelatedness of the many stories—the many narrative systems that we are as individuals; the many stories that, as individuals, we bring to our relationships; and the stories we find in our families and cultures. I will also suggest ways of listening to those stories and ways to hear more deeply and effectively inside an individual's story to discover the best way to help people live healthier stories. To that end I have included two chapters which focus more directly on ways of helping couples and families who are having problems. In those chapters I will suggest approaches to a variety of couple and family problems and the best strategies to help your couple and family deal with those problems.

Questions for Discussion

1. In what ways do we "live inside of stories"?
2. Who is responsible for your story (think beyond the obvious)?
3. Who or what launched you on your path to become a therapist?
4. What have been some major challenges in your story?
5. What would you change about your story going forward?

---

4   Lewis, T., Amini, F., & Lannon, R. (2001). *A General Theory of Love*, pp. 186–187.

CHAPTER TWO

The Story Within

CHAPTER SUMMARY AND LEARNING OBJECTIVE

Chapter 2 reviews the primary therapeutic approaches to treat individual clients. Special emphasis is placed on understanding personality development from both a causal as well as teleological perspective. The causal idea is that nature and nurture interact with each individual to create the traits and tendencies of character and personality. No doubt this is a true story, but is it the only story? The teleological story is that there is a type of internal blueprint that accounts for our particular interests and life trajectory. The notion that each human life is endowed with the ability to sense an inner direction has been a common human belief predating even Plato. It is essential for the clinician to grasp both the causal and teleological nature of human development in order to have a fuller understanding of the best approach to treat the story within each individual client.

The learning objective for this chapter is to fully grasp the causal and teleological perspectives in understanding the nature of human beings.

Your story didn't begin at your birth; it's not possible to know how far back your story goes. Some people and cultures believe that we choose not only when to be born but also the parents and culture that raise us. The idea behind this belief is that life is a classroom with the challenges we choose in order for our soul to grow and advance. Clearly, whatever the story, life *is* like a classroom, presenting many challenges and choices.

There are two important ideas in understanding human development: causal and teleological.[1] The causal idea is that nature and nurture interact with each other to create the traits and tendencies of our character and personality. No doubt this is a true story, but is it the only story? The teleological story describes human beings having an internal blueprint that accounts for our particular interests and life trajectory. The notion that each human life is endowed with the ability to sense an *inner* direction has been a common human belief predating even Plato.

---

[1] From the Greek "Telos" relating to the study of ultimate causes in nature or of actions in relation to their ends.

Alfred Adler, Carl Jung, Erik Erikson, and Abraham Maslow were among the first modern theorists to postulate what Carl Rogers termed the "actualization tendency"—the tendency for biological life to respond to an inner imperative to reach its potential. Adler talked about the concept of a "guiding fiction," the notion that even as children we begin to feel the pull of a particular story. If we are fortunate, the story unfolds throughout our life as it twists and turns through wrong directions and dead-ends until we emerge, hopefully, in a good place in our lives. Jung had a similar idea. He called it individuation. Individuation, in Jung's mind, was more of an inner journey. Through the course of our lives, we become more aware of our inner sense of Self and better able to handle the internal conflicts and confusion that compete with the unfolding of our journey toward wholeness. The term "Self" is Jung's teleological expression of this inner blueprint that guides our preferences and direction in life. Erikson found a similar word for life's goal. He called it integrity. Erikson was thinking of the less familiar and older idea of integrity not just as honesty but as a *holding together*. In the Navy, we used the term "water-tight integrity" to affirm that the ship didn't leak. Life *holds together* when we can reflect back on our lives with confidence that it was lived well, without too many leaks. Abraham Maslow's self-actualization is, perhaps, the best-known idea describing life's goal of realizing one's full potential. I used the term "fortunate" above because, according to Maslow, one must be fortunate enough to live in a time and place where one isn't preoccupied with survival and can enjoy the luxury of thinking about one's life and working to realize one's potential.

The concept of self-actualization must seem ridiculous to so many people just struggling to stay alive. For a fortunate few, reaching a state of self-actualization is achieving a confluence of *doing* and *being*—a state in which what one *does* is an extension of who one *is*. Again, this is a teleological perspective underscoring the possibility that one can experience a particular type of being which fits and is congruent with one's sense of self.

Clearly, the teleological perspective is at the heart of most religious thinking, as Rick Warren's *The Purpose Driven Life* (2011) attests. A fundamental tenant in theology is the notion that the soul is a unique spiritual endowment with the capacity to energize and direct one's journey. Interestingly, the teleological perspective also seems to show up in business literature from time to time. Steven Covey's *The Eighth Habit* (2005) is a good example. The subtitle of the book, *From Effectiveness to Greatness*, heralds Covey's encouragement to find one's authentic voice (or calling) and to help others to find theirs. In his view, enlightened business practice creates opportunity for individuals to experience their unique contribution and individual voice. Is this authentic voice the product of nature or nurture or is there something more? And what is that something more? As much as I would enjoy researching and reflecting on that question I'll simply state, for the purposes of this book, that it is useful and empowering to imagine that one's story exists as both the *push* of one's DNA and life experiences as well as the *pull* of that something more that belongs to each individual and can potentially influence the direction of his or her life, the *Soul's Code* (1997), as Jim Hillman called it.

Increasingly, psychologists look for an *evidence-based* approach to theories of personality and theories of counseling. Psychology, from this perspective, is a rigorous empirical science involving measurement, testing, and prediction. This is an important and valuable story. Testing truth is an essential human endeavor. The problem, of course, is that a statistical approach to understanding human behavior has limitations. Psychology has been forced to find other stories to explain human behavior—stories that can exist on a continuum between measurement and metaphor. The language of psychology is replete with shared metaphors. Terms such as "ego," "personality," "self-object," "identified patient," and "self-actualization" are all useful metaphors. Stories, not statistics, it turns out, are a much more interesting and useful language form with which to grasp human nature and potential. Therapists need to look more closely at some of these stories in order to get a better sense of the larger story of individuals and relationships.

I mentioned above that it's impossible to know exactly when an individual's story begins. Each of us is the product of the stories that went before. Practically speaking, I cannot think of a better introduction to an individual's story than that found in Dan Siegel's *The Developing Mind* (1999). The subtitle of his book says it all: *How relationships and the brain interact to shape who we are.* Siegel beautifully explains the interdependence of both nature and nurture:

> Therefore, caregivers are the architects of the way in which experience influences the unfolding of genetically preprogrammed but experience-dependent brain development. Genetic potential is expressed within the setting of social experiences, which directly influence how neurons connect to one another. Human connections create neuronal connections.[2]

In the quote above, Siegel describes the first *narrative system* of life: the story of parent and child. The parent contributes the DNA which sets the stage for the genetic unfolding. But it is the system of relatedness between parent and child, the "epigenetics," that drives the preprogrammed potential into actual neuronal connections. The interaction between the temperament of the infant and the temperament of the caregivers co-creates the experience-dependent brain development. This cooperation of infant and maternal/paternal interaction has been termed "attachment." And the nature of the story of attachment significantly influences the development of the individual's story for the rest of his or her life.

John Bowlby's trilogy, *Attachment* (1969), *Separation* (1973), and *Loss* (1980) revolutionized the study of human personality with his focus on the nature of maternal attachment as the most significant influence on human development. Mary Ainsworth, strongly influenced by Bowlby's work, developed the "strange situation" identifying four categories of attachment styles which substantially influence an individual's story. Initially, classic psychoanalysts objected to Bowlby's work, but the story of attachment is currently the most influential understanding of the developmental history of an individual. The significance of early attachments is recognized in other fields beyond psychology as well. In *The Stories We Live By*, Dan McAdams states,

> Secure attachment may nudge us in the direction of comedy and romance, insecure attachment, in the direction of tragedy and irony. ... By the time each of us reaches adolescence and adulthood, we are ready to create stories of a certain quality or type. By the time we think seriously about the meaning of our own lives, we may already

---

2   Siegel, D. (1999). *The Developing Mind*, p. 85.

be predisposed to create that meaning through the filtering glass of tragedy, comedy, irony, or romance.[3]

Before Bowlby and Ainsworth told their stories, Melanie Klein spoke of the relation of infant and mother in yet another system's narrative. Because of her background as a psychoanalyst, Klein used the familiar psychodynamic language of the ego and its objects (other people). Her object relations theory tells an imaginative story of how an infant might make sense of its very primitive world. Without the developed brain capacity to experience the actual person of the mother, all the infant can relate to are objects such as mouth, breast, hand, and so forth. A special problem exists when the infant is forced to deal with its own perplexing emotions. One of Klein's chief contributions to understanding human nature is her discussion of the infant's primitive defense of "splitting." Splitting external objects into all good or all bad (i.e., good breast and bad breast) is the infant's defense against the anxiety of its ambiguous experiences. Do adults, at times, also split experiences and people into all good or all bad? The answer isn't difficult, as the most recent "splitting" of parties and politics so clearly illustrates.

Harville Hendrix's *Getting the Love You Want* (2001) is a user-friendly application of Klein's object relations theory. Hendrix developed imago therapy for couples. The central tenant of that approach is an appreciation of the human tendency to *introject* the significant others (Kohut uses the term "self-objects")[4] of one's life. The introjected relationship with a significant other, usually mother or father, becomes the "imago" (image) of reenacted transference to one's present relationships. Understanding this dynamic for Hendrix (and other object relations theorists) is essential to understand the confusing and often conflicting dynamics of our interpersonal relationships.

Soren Kierkegaard tells another interesting story about human nature—an existential story. The problem with being a human mammal, according to Kierkegaard, is that we are both human and mammal. Being a mammal means that we are going to grow old and die. Being human means that we know it. "Angst" is the term Kierkegaard uses to describe the unavoidable anxiety of living with the simultaneous awareness of our amazing creative *possibility* and self-expression against the *necessity* of our mortality.[5] Erich Fromm tells a similar story. In *Escape from Freedom* (1941), Fromm warns that there is no escaping the anxiety of this existential dichotomy. It is the human dilemma to be able to conceptualize *infinite* possibilities for self-realization while living with *finite* limitations. This, the most fundamental *systems narrative* of life, is an extremely difficult story to live with. Fromm lists the many neurotic consequences of the all-too-common tendency to avoid thinking seriously about one's life and thus abandon one's freedom and potential to become fully human.

For Kierkegaard, the distinctive characteristic of human nature is response-ability. In his theological reflections, he suggests that human beings are endowed with the "ability to respond" to God, to each other, and to the earth. Not being responsible to our response-ability is a contradiction of human nature and the origin of manifold human problems. To be fully human is to be fully aware of our freedom to make choices as individuals. *The Courage to Create* (1975), according

---

3   McAdams, D. (1993). *The Stories We Live By*, p. 53.
4   Kohut discusses the concept of the self-object in *The Restoration of the Self* (1977).
5   Kierkegaard, S. (1844). *The Concept of Dread*.

to Rollo May, is the ability to embrace our finite existence and resist *The Denial of Death* (1973)[6] and the temptations, as Kierkegaard said, to be "tranquilized in trivia," in order to become an authentic Self, individuated, and self-actualized.

So far, the story *within* begins with our early attachments and object relations and continues with a brief visit to our essential, existential nature. Let's look a bit deeper into that story as Carl Jung invites us to consider the story with a view to our "internal systems narrative." Jung's colorful and fascinating tales of our internal drama have captured the imagination of Joseph Campbell in *Hero with a Thousand Faces* (1972), James Hillman in *The Soul's Code* (1997), and George Lucas in *Star Wars*. The *Star Wars* franchise celebrates Jung's imaginative writing about the symbols of the "collective unconscious" and the personification of archetypal images such as hero and heroine, the villain, the quest, the ordeal, and so forth. In film, we see ourselves. The engaging and powerful images on screen capture us and challenge us to experience our own internal story of loves, conflicts, and quests.

Jung offers a wealth of psychological vocabulary—a metaphorical language of the dynamics of the unconscious with which to plumb deeper insights into life's journey. Drawing heavily on mythological images, Jung explains that the archetypes of the collective unconscious[7] are those primordial imprinted images that inhabit the stories of peoples across time and geography. We find our own story narrated to us in the diverse characters of our personal unconscious. Eric Berne (1961) talked about our inner parent, adult, and child, but there are many others. The term "complex," for example, refers to the brain's tendency to accumulate emotionally laden associations of memory and perceptions that seem to have an autonomous life of their own. One finds oneself of two minds, the internal conflict between the dictates of one's inner parent and the demands of one's insistent inner child. This is the old superego vs. id story that Freud told; however, human beings have known that story since the beginning. In *The Stories We Live By* (1993), Dan McAdams tells us that

> The healing power of stories arises as a major theme in certain forms of psychotherapy, whose explicit therapeutic goal is the depathologizing of life. The development of a coherent life story is a major goal in these therapies. The analyst and the client seek to construct more adequate and vitalizing stories about the self. ... Some psychological problems and a great deal of emotional suffering stem from our failures to make sense of our lives through stories. Therapists help us revise our stories and produce a healing narrative of the self.

Another of Jung's contributions to understanding an individual's story is his development of the language of temperament. The subtitle of Jung's text on *Psychological Types* (1921) is *The Differentiation of Consciousness*. Jung constructed a language with which to describe how people differ in the way they see and respond to the world around them. Some people are more extraverted, while others are introverted; some perceive things concretely, while others perceive things symbolically; some make decisions analytically, others use subjective values; some like to be very organized, others prefer to be more flexible and spontaneous. Again, we

---

6   Becker, E. (1973). *The Denial of Death*.
7   Jung, C. (1959). *The Archetypes of the Collective Unconscious*.

see the complex interaction of two stories, DNA and the environment, working together to create a larger systems narrative of perception, response, and appetite.

When I attempt to explain personality type to people, I often clarify that it's important to appreciate that while an individual's temperament may lie on the *x axis*, the *y axis* depicts that individual's level of maturity. Temperament may be the *cards* that an individual is dealt, but his or her level of maturity dictates how the hand will be played. I frequently tell students that in order to anticipate a successful outcome in couple therapy you need to see three important qualities in your clients: a sufficient amount of motivation, insightfulness, and maturity. Clearly, it's hard to make progress if the motivation isn't there. An old joke in psychotherapy is "how many therapists does it take to change a light bulb?" The answer is "only one, but the light bulb has to want to change." Insightfulness is also important. Your clients need to be able to grasp what isn't working and acquire insight into how best to improve things. But it's your client's level of maturity that may be the most difficult challenge and the most important focus of your therapy. I'll explain.

Growth and maturity require doing hard things until they're not. A mature person manages difficult emotions until they are less difficult. He or she makes difficult choices and behaves responsibly even when it's hard. The ability to make wise, healthy, or loving choices in the face of difficult emotions is what Murray Bowen called "differentiation." Differentiation is acquired both internally and externally. Internal differentiation is the ability to differentiate thoughts and feelings and to be able to make good choices unencumbered by the challenging emotions of guilt or shame, or simple habit. External differentiation, then, is achieved when one can make healthy and wise *individual* decisions in the face of family or cultural pressure to uncritically comply. At one end of the *mature–immature* continuum are personality disorders. Alfred Adler was among the first modern psychologists to describe the defining qualities of mental/emotional disorders. Adler used the term "neurotic" to describe individuals who were straightjacketed by inflexibility, self-absorption, and self-protection. Neurotic safeguards, for Adler, are various styles of life created to protect a neurotic's fragile ego. "Mastery, excuses, and withdrawal" are the terms Adler used to explain how very immature people either want to control or dominate people, give away their power with habitual excuses, or withdraw from social contacts altogether. Karen Horney[8] identified the same three tendencies in people—efforts to take power from others, give their power to others, or abdicate their power altogether. She called these tendencies "neurotic trends."

Charles Dickens was a good story teller. His colorful description of various personality types and disorders are classic. In *Great Expectations*, for example, Miss Havisham spent the rest of her life encased in bitterness over having been jilted on her wedding day—a sad event, but checking out of life and staying in your wedding dress for years afterwards is taking neurotic rigidity to an extreme. Herman Melville could also tell a good story. People frequently got injured in the whaling industry, but Captain Ahab, having lost his leg to Moby Dick, clung tightly to his pride and hatred and, at the end, was literally tied to the white whale, the object of his megalomania.

At the other end of the mature–immature continuum is Maslow's *self-actualized*[9] individual. This is a person who is so practiced at making and living mature choices that those choices become second nature. Maslow described the self-actualized

8   Horney, K. (1945). *Our Inner Conflicts.*
9   Maslow, A. (1954). *Motivation and Personality.*

person as self-accepting, accepting of others, and accepting of what life has in store. It makes sense that if someone is self-accepting, he or she will be less needy of other people's approval and less concerned about their disapproval. Lacking these fears, one is freed to genuinely accept and authentically love others. Similarly, Julian Rotter[10] described a mature person as having an "internal locus of control"—again, the ability to be less dependent on other people's approval. Carl Rogers described a mature individual as a "fully functioning person."[11] A fully functioning person is more adaptable, more open to experiences, more self-aware, and more trusting in the ability to experience harmonious relations with others. According to M. Scott Peck, *The Road Less Traveled* (1988) requires accepting that life is difficult and the willingness to do the work: commitment to reality, the ability to delay gratification, taking responsibility, and balance. According to Peck, most people would prefer to avoid the hard facts of life and find ways to avoid working at their spiritual and emotional growth. Soren Kierkegaard had the same observation in his journal entry of 1837:

> There are many people who arrive at the result of their lives like school-boys; they cheat their teacher by copying the answer from the key in the arithmetic-book, without bothering to do the sums themselves.

Questions for Discussion

1. How might you apply the term "teleological" to your own story?
2. Would you be able to describe a personal experience with the concept of "calling"?
3. Review Erik Erikson's "Stages of the Life Cycle." Which stages do you feel you have completed adequately and which stages could use some additional work? Please explain.
4. What are the qualities of people who might be called self-actualized?
5. Can you think of anyone today who might be self-actualized?
6. Karen Horney explained the psychological defense of "splitting" in infants. Adults are also susceptible to using splitting as a psychological defense. Can you think of current illustrations?

---

10   Rotter, J. B. (1966). *Generalized Expectancies for Internal Versus External Control of Reinforcement.*
11   Rogers, C. (1961). *On Becoming a Person: A Therapist's View of Psychotherapy.*

CHAPTER THREE

Healing, Holding, Helping

The Work of Individual Psychotherapy

CHAPTER SUMMARY AND LEARNING OBJECTIVE

Chapter 3 emphasizes the principal tasks involved in therapy. The chapter explores the neural process involved in talk therapy and why talk therapy can be so effective in integrating and transforming neural pathways. This process is fundamental to the *healing* of traumatic memory and dissociative experience. Often clients present with grief, regret, and a sense of emptiness. *Holding* provides a consistent caring context in which clients can explore and work through these troubling experiences. Therapy, in this sense, is the work of providing that context. All therapy is potentially helpful. Often, *helping* our clients is simply providing some structure and direction so the problems can be more easily understood and solutions discovered.

The learning objective for this chapter is to understand the various ways in which therapy is effective in meeting the diverse needs of the client.

Individual psychotherapy was designed to help people find and follow that road less traveled. You, the therapist, are a companion on the journey. You are a guide on a mountain climb, or an undersea adventure. The guide knows the terrain and can provide a sense of security, direction, and encouragement. Clients in therapy face both the heights and depths of emotional work—work that may seem too frightening or difficult to do without the aid of an experienced guide. If, as I described above, you are one of the fortunate few in Maslow's hierarchy with the ability to integrate your *doing* with your *being*, you may feel *called* to do the work of therapy, or you may simply believe that you have what it takes to be a guide for the journey. There are three essential tasks in therapy: *healing*, *holding*, and *helping*.

Healing

The healing that takes place in psychotherapy is a systemic process impacting memory, emotion, cognition, behavior, and physical health. In working with individuals, talk therapy is the hub of a wheel with many spokes. According to Louis Cozolino (2002), in talk therapy

The combination of a goal-oriented and linear storyline, with verbal and nonverbal expressions of emotion, activates and utilizes processing of both left and right hemispheres, as well as cortical and subcortical processing. This simultaneous activation may be what is required for wiring and rewiring though the simultaneous or alternating activation of feelings, thoughts, behaviors, and sensations. The imprecision of stories may be a key to their success in the integration of neural systems with such diverse processing strategies.[1]

The spokes of the wheel, the many theoretical orientations and approaches that therapists use, serve to facilitate the process of "neural integration." Cozolino explains this process:

In most cases, the primary focus of psychotherapy is the integration of affect and cognition. Through the alternating activation of emotional and cognitive processes, the brain is able to interconnect neural networks responsible for those two functions. The various schools of therapy differ primarily in the emphasis they place on each of the human functions and the techniques they employ to regulate and integrate them.[2]

A simple description of this process for you to use with your clients is the chemical metaphor of adding a base ingredient to acid. In neural integration, the intensity of an emotional memory or experience is accessed, integrated, and somewhat neutralized. The term "catharsis" describes the access and release of emotion. Catharsis may be profound or subtle, but the net effect is experienced as a physiological release of tension. People feel better. One can have a cathartic experience by going to the movies, reading a good book, or talking with a friend, but the managed and directed process of talk therapy by an experienced clinician can have profound and lasting emotional and even physical benefits.

Three psychiatrists, Lewis, Amini, and Lannon,[3] remind us of the connection of psychology and physiology and underscore the important role talk therapy plays in facilitating healing:

The mind-body clash has disguised the truth that psychotherapy is physiology. When a person starts therapy, he isn't beginning a pale conversation; he is stepping into a somatic state of relatedness. Evolution has sculpted mammals into their present form: they become attuned to one another's evocative signals and alter the structure of one another's nervous systems. Psychotherapy's transformative power comes from engaging and directing these ancient mechanisms. Therapy is a living embodiment of limbic processes as corporeal as digestion or respiration. Without the psychologic unity limbic operations provide, therapy would indeed be the vapid banter some people suppose it to be.

---

1   Cozolino, L. (2002). *The Neuroscience of Psychotherapy*, p. 170.
2   Cozolino, L. (2004). *The Making of a Therapist*, p. 32.
3   Lewis, T., Amini, F., & Lannon, R. (2000). *A General Theory of Love*, p. 168.

Clients regularly tell me in everyday language that "getting things off their chest" helps them to feel lighter, sleep better, have more energy, and feel more optimistic. The quotes above have been especially helpful to me. I used to wonder how simply talking about a problem or how someone feels could help them to feel better. I now have a better understanding of the neurophysiology of talk therapy—how and why it works. It isn't simply vapid banter. When therapy works, when people do feel better, it is because of the quality of connection that facilitates the creation of new neural pathways that transform the physiology of the brain. Effective therapy helps people to heal.

Holding

In addition to healing, therapy requires *holding*. We hold our clients with the quality of our care, compassion, and consistency. We provide a safe, consistent, and reliable environment in which clients feel encouraged to be open about their struggles, practice being vulnerable, and learn to tolerate difficult emotions. In classic psychoanalytic language, a therapist "holds the frame"—the ground rules and ethical boundaries that maintain confidentially and professionalism in treatment.

Donald Winnicott, an English psychoanalyst and pediatrician, emphasized that the quality of care provided by the mother for her infant was the foundation of a child's early experience of well-being. Adequate attunement of mother to infant provided the security and assurance of being known and valued. Just so, in therapy, the therapist creates a "holding environment" in which the client feels secure and valued. According to Winnicott, "A correct and well-timed interpretation in an analytic treatment gives a sense of being held that is more real than if a real holding or nursing had taken place."[4]

We *hold* our clients as they struggle to make sense of loss, abandonment, and betrayal. We become the temporary *safe haven* and secure base when it seems to them that their world is falling apart. We create an environment of acceptance and security through the agonizing months of recovery from trauma and the reconstruction of a shattered life.

The humanistic, *person-centered* approach of Carl Rogers defined the therapeutic qualities necessary to create a *holding environment*. Over time, as clients experience unconditional positive regard, empathic listening, and genuineness, their hearts and lives begin to open to the possibility of feeling safe, feeling interesting, feeling valued.

> People do come to therapy unable to love and leave with that skill restored. But love is not only an end for therapy; it is also the means whereby every end is reached.[5]

Rollo May, an existential psychologist, uses the Greek term *agape* to underscore that love in the context of therapy, as Roger's said, is the ability to offer unconditional caring and acceptance. In other words, you give your clients your best. How can that happen?

---

4   Winnicott, D. W. (1965). *The Family and Individual Development.*
5   Lewis, T., Amini, F., & Lannon, R. (2000). *A General Theory of Love*, p. 169.

Have courage. You have your training and supervision. You know your ethical standards. You understand the importance of doing no harm. The scary part for many therapists is exactly what I quoted above—stepping into a somatic state of relatedness. That means allowing yourself to step into another's shoes, to try to imagine what it must be like to be that person and to experience what they are experiencing. There have many times in therapy that I found that I could not say anything that didn't sound trite or insensitive. The enormity of what my patient was feeling left me speechless. Over time, I came to realize that not knowing what to say was a good thing. It meant that I was doing my job. The word compassion comes from the Latin root "to suffer with." I couldn't think of anything to say because I was inside of that person's story, suffering with them. Of course, it's impossible to genuinely feel what another is feeling, but I could feel my own feelings and what I might be experiencing inside of that person's story. Try not to be afraid when that happens. You are doing your job. Remember that your task is not to fix the person or the story. You are simply asked to care. The closer you can get to another's story, the more that person will feel felt and cared about. This is the central narrative system in therapy, the quality of the relationship you have with your client.

You will suffer in this profession. You will work hard, and you won't get rich. If you're doing your job well, you will be adequately compensated. You will earn a decent living, but your principal incentive isn't what you'll earn but the opportunity to be who you are. If you do well in this profession it is because you have been called to it. I had a short dream when I was in school to become a therapist. I was standing at the sink about to do the dishes. I looked through the soapy water and noticed that the dishes were made of glass and were all broken. The message of the dream was clear. I realized that if I were to presume to reach into people's lives, I had better be careful. Broken dishes can cut.

The idea of a "calling" is very old. It can be described as an inner knowing, a sense of direction, a pull toward having and becoming an authentic Self. The existential thinking of Otto Rank, Erich Fromm, Rollo May, Victor Frankl, and especially Soren Kierkegaard come close to describing the felt sense of rightness when one is able to become that Self. Some people ascribe that pull to God or to an experience of the "numinous." For others, it's simply what they want to do or who they want to become. In either case, to survive in the profession, it's good to know that there is, in the language of recovery, "a power greater than yourself" that is guiding you on your journey. Your suffering will be more than the times that people abruptly leave therapy without telling you why, or the person who misinterprets something you've said, or the client who talks about you negatively to others. These, unavoidably, come with the profession. The real suffering happens when, after a time, you begin to feel pressed down by how hard life is, the unfairness, the selfishness, the enormity of pain in the world. If you're doing your job, you will become more vulnerable, more porous. It will be harder to carry on small talk. There will be movies you can't watch and television shows that feel too much like work or hit too close to home. You'll need faith to keep going.

Your faith is in the remarkable ability people have to heal and recover. Your faith will be in the power of caring and the transformative power of your therapeutic skills. Your faith may be in God's guidance or the transcendent power of love. You will need your faith to keep you going when you're working with a very injured client. Some clients have had such traumatic lives that they have necessarily built up a very solid wall of self-protection. Over time, your calming confidence and compassion will work wonders. I love what Jeff Kottler reports in his wonderful book *On Being a Therapist*. He relates a portion of a conversation he had with a client who told him that there were many things about therapy that were helpful, but that the most helpful thing was his faith in her. "You believed in me," she said, "and I believed in you, and eventually I came to believe in myself." I think Jeff's client would agree with the notion that she had felt "held" in therapy.

The emphasis of existential therapy is to create a context where one is held in a creative space in which to search for meaning and discover the freedom, response-ability, and courage to be one's *authentic self*. The core consideration in both the humanistic and existential approach to therapy is that which promotes the actualizing tendency described above. Erikson reminded us that not everyone accomplishes each of the developmental tasks required to be fully actualized throughout his or her lifespan, but the potential remains throughout. The challenge for therapists is to help individuals "unlock" these sometimes-hidden capacities.

Erikson called the first development task of life "trust vs. mistrust." In this early stage of life, a person comes to believe that life may be somewhat predictable and benevolent—or not. If the caring an infant receives is adequate, the infant may develop essential trust. If the caring is sketchy and unpredictable, an infant may struggle with lifelong difficulties trusting. Winnicott talked about the infant's need for a blanket or teddy bear to serve as a *transitional object* in the process of weaning one's dependency on the mother's presence. The therapist volunteers to be that transitional object for her client. In object relations language, the therapist becomes a significant but temporary "self-object" with whom the client repairs or develops a positive self-image. Through the stabilizing and fortifying influence of therapy, the client finds the internal resources, ego strengths, and life skills with which to move forward. The therapeutic alliance becomes a resourceful, if not life changing, chapter in the client's story.

Helping

Helping people with their problems is the third important task in psychotherapy. Obviously, the nature of the problem dictates the nature of the therapy. Hopefully, all approaches to therapy are helpful in some ways. People seek therapy when they're not happy. When people aren't happy with their relationships, with their work, with their children, with their lives, you'll get a call. People will complain that they need to change their behaviors, change how they think about things, or change how they feel. Arnold Lazarus (1995) has created the acronym BASIC ID. In his acronym, Lazarus describes the seven important domains of human concerns: **B**ehavior, **A**ffect, **S**ensation, **I**magery, **C**ognition, **I**nterpersonal relationships, and **D**rugs and biology. According to Lazarus, each domain interacts with and affects other domains. We know that our thoughts, feelings, and behaviors are all connected and that making changes in one area affects the other two. Lazarus wisely expands this concept of interconnectedness to include our physical sensations and biology, how we experience our relationships, as well as our imaginal life—our memories, dreams, and how we picture ourselves. These domains of mutual interaction will emerge individually or in in clusters in therapy, and the core concept of cognitive-behavioral therapy is that focusing attention in one area of one's life will affect the others—a fundamental narrative system. One important area that Lazarus neglected is what Barbara Ingram has termed the "spiritual domain." According to Ingram, "The term 'spiritual' applies to a wide variety of experiences, beliefs, and activities. Clients who are coping with death, moral dilemmas, and blocks to creativity often benefit from a spiritual focus."[6] Ingram goes on to describe conversations and methods to help clients connect with their spiritual resources. For Ingram, Lazarus' acronym becomes BASIC SIDS. I like Ingram's book for its extremely practical approach to case formulation and treatment ideas. Ingram lists 30 potential client problems and skillfully integrates various strategies from a variety of clinical approaches that will best fit and treat the client's problems.

It was Albert Ellis (2005)[7] who developed the ABCDE model, reiterating that the emotional **C**onsequence of an **A**ctivating event is dependent on one's **B**elief about the event. In cognitive therapy, a **D**isputing intervention—challenging your client's cognitive distortions, automatic negative thoughts, and disruptive core beliefs—will eventually help them to produce a new **E**motional outcome. Obviously, this formula is at the heart of all self-help books. And, obviously, it works—some of the time. Success in CBT depends on the client's willingness to learn and rehearse skills. Here again, the therapist may encounter the three compromising challenges of change: motivation, maturity, and insightfulness. Change is frequently difficult and new ways of thinking, feeling, and behaving require practice. The best types of self-help books include recommendations for how to practice making those changes.

Sometimes, helping your clients isn't difficult. They need advice on how to approach launching their 24-year-old son still living at home, or help with a specific decision, or a place where they can brainstorm ideas about dealing with in-laws, or finances, or household chores. In crisis situations, on the other hand, helping can be extremely difficult. Deciding whether to divorce, or dealing with a family death or tragedy, the loss of employment, or internet drama can be a real crisis in the life of a family. In these situations, your clarity and calming presence can be extremely helpful. Remember that your understanding of the integrated narrative systems of human experience will inform your assessment of your clients' problems. That assessment will determine your treatment plan, your goals, and your helping strategies. You and your client live inside of the stories that your brains are telling you about your experience together. You are both searching for the story that best fits your client's problem and a way of conceptualizing the best narrative for progress. Recall that

> Narrative storytelling is the primary model humans possess for the sequential and meaningful integration of human action. Narratives are a vehicle for explaining behavior and defining both the social and private selves. Narratives are emotionally meaningful, causally linked sequences of actions and consequences that aid in the organization, maintenance, and evaluation of behavior.[8]

You are a professional listener. You listen with your ears, your mind, and your heart. Your training has equipped you to listen to your client's story more deeply

---

6   Ingram, B. (2006). *Clinical Case Formulations.*
7   Ellis, A. (2005). *Rational Emotive Behavioral Therapy* is the culmination of lifelong work as a cognitive-behavioral therapist. In the mid-1950s Ellis first introduced the ABCDE model.
8   Cozolino, L. (2002). *The Neuroscience of Psychotherapy*, p. 166, referring to the work of K. Oatley (1992) and R. Fivush (1994).

and effectively because you have been educated in the five main genres in which psychological stories take place, the *psychodynamic*, the *humanistic/existential*, the *cognitive* and *behavioral*, the *systemic*, and the *medical/biological* genres. The individual story is enlarged and more fully grasped when it is understood in the larger context of the human story. Your ear picks up the background of the story and detects, with your internal compass, the direction the story is headed. Even though you can imagine this story from a larger perspective, you remain respectful of your client's own individual life and experience. And so you help to integrate and elaborate your client's story in a manner that helps your client not only to *feel felt* but to see renewed possibilities for the direction the story may take. Frequently, the most effective intervention, from an *attuned* therapist, is a simple sentence or a single word that helps the client to see her path more clearly. Your professional education not only supplies you with an ability to hear the deeper contexts of a client story but also the language in which to capsulize the story in brief. Talking with my client, Janice, I simply stated, "You're feeling stuck." "Yes, that's exactly it," she exclaimed, and began to weep. Certainly, not a profound intervention, but she felt "heard" and, for the moment, less alone. Offering a simple word or sentence when a client needs to feel truly heard comes from careful attention and thorough knowledge of the many narrative systems with which to hear, more clearly, what the story is saying and what the story wants. Lewis, Amini, and Lannon (2000) describe the therapist who is able to allow the process of limbic resonance to attain that quality of attunement:

> If a listener quiets his neocortical chatter and allows limbic sensing to range free, melodies begin to penetrate the static of anonymity. Individual tales of reactions, hopes, expectations, and dreams resolve into themes. Stories about lovers, teachers, friends, and pets echo back and forth and coalesce into a handful of motifs. As the listener's resonance grows, he will catch sight of what the other sees inside that personal world, start to sense what it feels like to live there.

The narrative system we will explore next will be *the story between*—the system of relatedness in couples. In the next chapter we will look at the dynamics, the limbic processes, of attraction and attachment. In addition, we will delve more deeply into the nature of interpersonal relationships to show how two individual stories combine to make a third, and how that third story becomes larger than the sum of its parts.

Questions for Discussion

1. Have you ever experienced catharsis? How might you describe the feeling in your body?
2. How is therapy different from talking with a close friend?
3. Do you recall the feeling of being emotionally held as an adult?
4. What can be frightening about allowing yourself to genuinely care about a client?
5. How will you repair yourself after an especially intense therapy session?

CHAPTER FOUR

Love Stories

CHAPTER SUMMARY AND LEARNING OBJECTIVE

Chapter 4 introduces the work of Lewis, Amini, and Lannon in *A General Theory of Love*. According to these authors, limbic resonance, limbic regulation, and limbic revision account for the dynamics of attraction and the neural physiology of stable and healthy relationships. The chapter also reviews John Bowlby and Mary Ainsworth's development of attachment theory and the role that attachment and reenactment play in damaging or healing relationships. Healthy conflict is important in relationships. People that prize growth understand that differences are as important as similarities in maintaining a dynamic, interesting, and growth-producing relationship. The chapter explains why conflict exists in relationships, explains why it is important to understand the nature and background of conflict, and points to the steps needed to grow from conflict.

> *The learning objective for this chapter is to understand the limbic processes at work in the dynamics of attraction and in establishing and maintaining attachment in relationships.*

Attraction and Attachment

The most powerful narrative system on earth, the one most written and sung about, is love.

Love can keep us alive. That isn't simply a beautiful romantic sentiment. According to Drs. Lewis, Amini, and Lannon, it is a neurological fact. In *A General Theory of Love,* they use the terms *limbic resonance, limbic regulation,* and *limbic revision* to describe the biological benefits and essential nature of human attachment. Stories of love and attachment may be the most profound stories in the galaxy of narrative systems:

> Because loving is a reciprocal physiologic influence, it entails a deeper and more literal connection than most realize. Limbic regulation affords

lovers the ability to modulate each other's emotions, neurophysiology, hormonal status, immune function, sleep rhythms, and stability. If one leaves on a trip, the other may suffer insomnia, a delayed menstrual cycle, a cold that would have been fought off in the fortified state of togetherness. The neurally ingrained attractors of one lover warp the emotional virtuality of the other, shifting emotional perceptions—what he feels, sees, knows. When somebody loses his partner and says a part of him is gone, he is more right that he thinks. A portion of his neural activity depends on the presence of that other living brain. (p. 207–208)

I don't dislike country music. In fact, I was listening to Patsy Cline the other day and it seemed to me that most of her songs were either about the loss of love or the longing for love. I don't presume to characterize any music genre, but I can't help thinking that a disproportionate amount of attachment issues arise in country and western ballads. Maybe I'm not being fair. There are certainly many illustrations of attachment issues showing up in other types of music.

For example, I remember when the Righteous Brothers sang,

> *You're my soul, my life's inspiration, all I've got to get me by—without you, baby, what good am I?*

"Soul & Inspiration," The Righteous Brothers

I used to think that was the theme song of people with dependent personality disorder, and I sometimes found myself wanting to say, "Dude, get a life!" But after reading *A General Theory of Love*, I'm much less critical of the Righteous Brothers song. While it may not be great poetry, one can certainly sympathize with the pain of the loss of a significant attachment. The song illustrates what John Bowlby[1] referred to as the "protest stage" of separation anxiety. "I am alone and afraid," squeals the baby chick, the puppy, the human infant, or a Righteous Brother separated from its attachment object. Countless stories and songs have been written about the pain of separation and the loss of love. This is something that all human beings seem to understand and feel; when put into words or music, it resonates at a deep level for most of us. Separation is painful and frightening because attachment is *essential* for survival. If a four-year-old is briefly separated from her parents at Disneyland, for instance, her screams of terror might seem unwarranted to an adult. But this young mammal, separated from her protective pack, does not know, at a deeply instinctive, biological level, that she will not be eaten! Her screams alert her caregivers to her whereabouts and soon bring reassuring rescue. Other adult mammals are alerted to one of their own kind in distress and will respond if her parents aren't immediately present. This is human survival, and when people in love call each other "baby" or some other cute endearment, it signifies the essential deal that lovers make to be honest about their vulnerability and their need for attachment.

Enter conflict. Conflict exists because people compete to survive, and attachment is essential for survival. When attachment is threatened people get scared and angry. Fear and anger create defenses and defensiveness leads to conflict. Consequently, healthy attachments are not easy to achieve. In fact, the very reasons

1   Bowlby, J. (1973). *Separation: Anxiety and Anger*, pp. 21–22.

one is attracted to his or her partner is, paradoxically, the other side of the coin from many of the reasons for conflict. I'll explain.

Attachment Styles

In her research with children, Mary Ainsworth, a student of John Bowlby, found that when mothers provide adequate and consistent care, children experience mom as a safe haven from which to explore their world. Inadequate or inconsistent care may result in children becoming easily upset, clingy, and inconsolable on the one hand, or insecure, avoidant, and self-protective on the other. These attachment patterns regularly persist into adult life, yielding relationship styles that Harville Hendrix has called fusers and isolators.[2] Fusers may have felt pushed away or disconnected from caring relationships as children and crave close connections as adults. Isolators may have been over-protected, over-controlled, and smothered as children and are afraid of too much closeness as adults. Hendrix's observations coincide with my own. It often seems that one person in a relationship tends to be anxious about losing connection with his or her partner and the other person tends to be anxious about losing independence—the connection to themselves. Here is another interesting observation: the two types of people tend to be attracted to each other.

Marriage therapists see a great deal of diversity in the reasons why people are attracted to each other. But they also find some very consistent patterns. It is very illuminating to discover these patterns in relationships and to understand how, like it or not, our upbringing does affect how we relate to a partner. Obviously, these attachment patterns are not often clear-cut. And even people with a happy childhood and secure attachments will feel insecure, disconnected, or avoidant at times. It wasn't just the Righteous Brothers that had problems with insecure and co-dependent attachments. The Four Tops sang about attachment anxiety in their hit song "Sugar Pie, Honey Bunch":

> *Snap your finger, wink your eye, I'm running to you; tied to your apron strings, there's nothing I can do.*

Knowing a few things about human nature can sure ruin your enjoyment of the "oldies." I was quoting from one of these oldies in class when one of my students said, "Dr. Buckley, I think you need to update your iTunes."

Early in life, it seems to us that the harder we work to be good or acceptable or delightful, the more love we experience. This is a childish equation, but one that most people learn as they grow up and continues to affect them as adults. Obviously and unfortunately some children learn early to discard that equation. For them, love is unpredictable, inadequate, and impossible to trust.

For the unloved, there is no security or significance except in one's own efforts to isolate or dominate. In either case, adults work to acquire love, to hold on to love, or to protect themselves from the vulnerability of love. Love is complex because, on the one hand, it entices us with the possibility of a child-like experience of unconditional love, a love that is given freely, a love that nurtures our deepest needs

---

2   Hendrix, H. (1988). *Getting the Love You Want*, p. 21.

for security and significance. On the other hand, adult love involves commitment and sacrifice—the work of safeguarding and nurturing the well-being of another.

Love is complex and confusing because it requires the difficult task of managing the paradox of balancing concern for another with concern for oneself. This paradox of conflicting strivings (a most essential narrative system) provides the vital context in which human love is tested, stretched, and deepened into mature love.

To understand this process, it's important to grasp the less obvious reasons why we are attracted to our partners. Those reasons come primarily from differences in our temperaments, attachment styles, and the peculiar dynamics of "reenactment." Temperament is inherited and modified by our attachment to our parents. Reenactment is the tendency to be attracted to a person who has the ability to put us in touch with familiar feelings. You, the therapist, must understand the role that personality style, attachment, and reenactment play in relationships. Each of these dynamics surfaces in attraction on the one hand and in confusion and conflict on the other. They are two sides of the same coin. You must understand the role that each of these dynamics play in the relationship in order to explain, illuminate, and direct the efforts of a couple to learn and grow from each other.

> When our earliest overtures for comfort were regularly welcomed, we probably learned the advantages of turning to others to soothe our distress; when such early overtures evoked rejection, we probably learned the necessity of concealing our distress from others whenever possible. Such primal lessons about self and others are learned—remembered, represented, internalized—as they are enacted. Later rather than being recognized with a sensation of recollection, these hard-to-verbalize representations are recognized—generally by third parties, if at all—mainly as they are enacted.[3]

These "remembered, represented, internalized, and enacted" memories are what Harville Hendrix refers to as an imago in his popular text *Getting the Love You Want* (1988). I asked Janice why she thought her husband was attracted to her. "I don't know," she replied. I knew that she wasn't simply being modest. She truly had no idea. After 27 years of marriage, she ought to have known. It's sad, but not uncommon. Far too many couples have no idea. Apart from the standard "we have similar values," "she was nice looking," "I thought he would make a good father," few couples seem to have any grasp of the depths of their attraction. The reasons above aren't bad reasons, but there's more to why we make the choice to spend our life with someone. Something about being with this person feels familiar. One can be conscious of that feeling and say something like, "I feel like I have known you all of my life." But often the sense of familiarity is under the surface; only later do people see the resemblance to significant people from their past. The logic of this attraction is in the brain's tendency to attempt to repair deficits or psychic wounds from earlier in life. "We marry our homework," I once found myself saying.

The brain seems to be interested in growth. In *A General Theory of Love* (2000), the authors discuss the brain's tendency to seek out limbic resonance (connection to another), limbic regulation (a stable relationship), and limbic revision (mental and emotional growth). The authors go on to say that the brain has an uncanny

---

3   Wallin, D. (2007). *Attachment in Psychotherapy*, p. 122–123.

radar for that person with whom, for better or worse, the brain can undertake the task of reenactment.

I discuss more about reenactment later. For now, Janice believes that Steven loves her, but she doesn't know why. I asked Steven if he knew why Janice loved him. "My striking good looks," he replied, and they both laughed. They were genuinely puzzled about why I was asking the question and perhaps even more puzzled that neither of them had thought very much about the answer. Why is it important for Steve and Janice to know why they love and are loved? The answer is so that they can consciously participate in the growth that their love can produce. Steven and Janice are different people. They have different temperaments, different appetites, and different backgrounds and baggage. They need to understand that those differences need not be a source of ongoing irritation and conflict. In fact, the differences are a huge factor in why they were attracted to each other to begin with. But they need to understand how to manage those differences. This requires three critical tasks. They need to (1) become aware of who they are as individuals, their strengths and work areas; (2) learn how to share that information safely; and (3) be able to negotiate their values, ways of being, and appetites. Those tasks form the bedrock of a stable and growing relationship. Being romantic and affectionate, enjoying each other, having fun, and managing life together complete the picture. This is where you, the therapist, can help them with the insight and skills they need to reach those goals.

Questions for Discussion

1. How would you characterize your own experience with attachment?
2. What other songs do you know that address the ups and downs of attachment?
3. What role do personality types play in attraction?
4. Can you describe the process of reenactment? Can you illustrate what that might look like with a couple?
5. What does Hendrix mean by the term imago? How does that concept figure into your therapy?

CHAPTER FIVE

Stories of Temperament, Attraction, and Negotiating Perceptions

CHAPTER SUMMARY AND LEARNING OBJECTIVE

Chapter 5 attempts to answer the question of why couples are attracted to each other and how to deal with the differences implicit in attraction. I discuss the Myers–Briggs Type Indicator as a useful method of understanding personality and personality differences. In addition to those differences, the dynamics of "reenactment" play an important role in attraction. Harvell Hendrix and others discuss the theory of object relations—the tendency, in a relationship, to be attracted to a person who puts one in touch with familiar emotions from growing up. The brain's agenda in this form of attraction is to reenact childhood experiences with the possibility of obtaining new emotional outcomes. In successful relationships, couples explore the deeper logic of their attraction to each other, learn to value differences, and work together to precipitate healing and growth. To achieve this advanced level of relationship, couples learn to manage defensive emotions in order to have increasingly open and vulnerable communication, in which different perceptions are valued and negotiated. In this way, two become a larger and more dynamic *one*.

The learning objective for this chapter is to understand the connection between attraction, attachment, and the dynamics of reenactment.

Temperament

Isabel Briggs-Myers with her mother Katharine Briggs used the personality concepts developed by Carl Jung to create the means to assess differences in people's temperaments. The Myers–Briggs Type Indicator uses 160 questions to determine whether you tend to be more extraverted or introverted, whether you perceive things more concretely or symbolically, whether you tend to make decisions analytically or tend to use more subjective values, and whether you prefer things to be decided and managed or more flexible and spontaneous. The MBTI has been greatly refined over the years and may be obtained from Consulting Psychologist Press in Palo Alto, California.

I took the MBTI for the first time in 1977 and began using it in marital and premarital counseling that same year. Since that time, I have scored hundreds of MBTIs. I have found it to be a very effective way of looking at differences between people and an aid to understanding the variety and complexity of their relationships. I especially appreciate the MBTI as a means to help people better understand themselves, their ways of expressing and experiencing love, managing life, and dealing with conflicts. The MBTI is also often used in academic and occupational contexts as an aid to finding one's career path or best fit in a business organization.

Over many years of clinical use, I have noticed some regularly occurring patterns in interpersonal relationships. I've noticed, for example, that it's rare for people with identical temperaments to be attracted to each other. Totally opposite temperaments don't seem to be attracted to each other either. These types of relationships exist but they are not the norm. It is more common for couples to share two of the four temperamental continuums in common and have two different. People tend to be attracted to a balance of similarities and differences. This balance of similarities and differences seems to provide many couples with the benefits of familiarity sufficient to establish rapport and negotiate values and lifestyle, while also providing challenges for diversity and growth. An ideal relationship is neither too boring nor too challenging.

Interestingly, people seem to be attracted to wholeness as much (if not more) than to happiness. If people simply wanted to be happy it seems reasonable that they would look for someone who has an identical temperament and is easy to live with. But that virtually never happens. It's true that if people were too similar there would be very little work involved, very little stretching, and very little conflict—but also very little growth. So, whether consciously or unconsciously, people tend to be attracted to differences as much as to similarities—hence, the existence of marriage counselors.

Reenactment

Reenactment is the very common phenomenon of discovering that the delightfully *familiar* feeling one has with the person who seems "exactly right" is due to the brain's ability to recognize similar *familiar* feelings from childhood. In other words, something about our relationship with this present person feels similar to important relationships we've had in the past. Here again, it's useful to refer to Hendrix's *Getting the Love You Want*.

Hendrix isn't saying that we marry people who resemble our mothers or fathers physically or even psychologically. He's saying that we are attracted to relationship *dynamics* that are already familiar to us. Like so many other unconscious dynamics, that could be good news or bad news. The "right" person will often put us in touch with what we felt earlier in life, in our relationship with our mother or father. These are extremely powerful relationships that are strongly imprinted in our neural pathways. This implicit or automatic imprinting process creates a personal "schema" or mental/emotional outlook. Our schema consists of a system of beliefs and expectations that influence our perceptions and interpretations of our experiences and relationships. Louis Cozolino puts it this way:

> Attachment schemas are implicit memories that are known without
> being thought. Because they are stored in the architecture of the social

brain as predictions of the behaviors of others, they "create" the people we meet and unconsciously guide our reactions to them. Early attachment schemas persist into adulthood, impacting our choice of partners and the quality of our relationships. Their impact goes beyond the ability to shape our relationships; they also influence our emotional life, immunological functioning, and experience of self.[1]

Hendrix encourages couples to understand that reenactment happens. In good relationships (Hendrix calls them *conscious* marriages) people discover that the person they love can bring out both the best and the worst qualities in them. The traditional marriage vow, "for better or for worse," seems to acknowledge that inevitable dynamic in marriage. Because, in so many ways, the relationship is familiar and because the brain does what brains do, we attach present experiences to past memories. Mostly for survival, the brain tends to make very quick connections and associations with past experiences. Those significant and sometimes life-saving associations provide additional protection from harmful situations, opportunities for the brain to learn new adaptive skills, and an extra incentive to seek out protective and meaningful attachments. But those same past/present associations the brain makes so automatically and effortlessly can also be very disturbing. The emotional memory of those old experiences can be triggered by present contexts and intensify one's emotional reaction. Here again, Lewis, Amini, and Lannon have a very picturesque description of the process of reenactment:

> People target the mates who mesh with their own minds, and they do so with the speed and precision that our smartest smart bombs are not sufficiently intelligent to envy ... Most people will choose misery with a partner their limbic brain recognizes over the stagnant pleasure of a "nice" relationship with someone their attachment mechanism cannot detect.[2]

Just so, Patsy Cline sings "He gives me ... love that ... I never got from you. He loves me too. ... Why can't he be you?"

Memory

When we talk about pleasant memories, we often describe the images in our mind, recall the pleasant emotions associated with the experience, and, at times, even feel the physical sensations associated with the memory—the smells, the tastes, the sounds, and so forth. In this sense, a memory can be complete with images, emotions, and sensations. We can have partial memories as well. Sometimes we remember an image without much emotion or sensation. And, interestingly, we can also have "emotional memories." Emotional memory occurs when a present experience is intensified by the emotional connection with our past experiences. There may not be any visual images of the past, but the brain recalls the experience and creates mental associations. Again, this may be a pleasant experience or an even more intensely painful one.

---

1   Cozolino, L. (2006). *The Neuroscience of Human Relationships*, p. 148.
2   Lewis, T., Amini, F., & Lannon, R. (2000). *A General Theory of Love*, p. 161.

Lulled in the countless chambers of the brain, our thoughts are linked by many a hidden chain; awake but one, and lo, what myriads rise!

Alexander Pope

There is not a man living who has not, some time in his life, admitted that memory was as much a curse as a blessing.

F. A. Durivage

Many of our most enjoyable and painful experiences occur when we were young and more vulnerable to the joys and pains of our attachment to our parents. Consequently, as an adult, being with a person who is very emotionally important to you will sometimes trigger emotions that are similar to emotions you felt growing up. Again, for better or for worse, whether we like it or not, we are very vulnerable to the people we love. So unless one is very defensive and guarded, it is very easy to experience the phenomenon of reenactment. That is to say, from time to time, we may be vulnerable to feeling small, feeling needy, and sometimes feeling frightened. Our partners have the uncanny ability to trigger our greatest joys but also to ignite our deepest fears, our repeated negative experiences, our traumas, our damaged self-esteem, and our unfinished work. That feels bad, but it can potentially be very good.

I'll explain. We give the person we love a great deal of power. We give them the power to make us feel important, to feel loved, to feel joy, to look forward to the future. We also give them the power to hurt us, betray us, abandon us, and make us feel worthless. We may argue that we shouldn't give them that much power, but when you're in love, you lose that argument.

My wife had an inscription etched on the inside of my wedding ring. It reads, "Wonderful and Terrifying." When we give someone the power to wound us, we also give them the power to help us to heal, wonderfully, not just from present wounds, but from past hurts as well. The key to that depth of healing is the ability to be vulnerable with each other.

And the key to vulnerability is trust. Ideally, lovers give the other permission to wound them. When lovers, who have that power, choose not to wound each other, trust is built.

Clearly building and securing trust is a very delicate process. More about that below.

Choices

When we ask our partner to make loving choices, choices that significant people in our lives growing up may not have made, two things happen. First, we have the opportunity to experience a quality and quantity of love that penetrates deep into our soul. This happens over time with increasing trust, vulnerability, intimacy, and attachment. Second, because, as we have seen, the person we are attracted to will typically express and experience love differently than we do, their choice to love us will require effort. Genuine love always does. When our lover makes an effort to love us in ways that are especially meaningful to us, we experience our own value. This, then, is a double blessing. In the presence of genuine love, one not only feels loved, but also valued. This is love that transcends the merely biological need for attachment. It is the love that originates in the human spirit. It is what the Greeks referred to as *agape*. Rollo May referred to the term agape as the joining of will and care, the unconditional love that arises from the human capacity to participate in the divine love of the creator. The relationship that is characterized by this quality of love is not just therapeutic, it's miraculous. Saint Paul described this kind of love:

> *Love is patient, love is kind, and is not jealous; Love does not brag and is not arrogant, does not act unbecomingly; it does not seek its own, is not provoked, does not take into account a wrong suffered, does not rejoice in unrighteousness, but rejoices with the truth; bears all things, believes all things, hopes all things, endures all things. Love never fails.*

I Corinthians 13:4–8 New American Standard Version

Clearly this kind of love is difficult. Every couple has heard the cliché that marriage requires hard work, but too few couples know what that means. The hard work isn't just putting up with another person although, sadly, that may be too true for many people. The hard work is genuinely loving them. I also like Scott Peck's definition of love: "the will to extend oneself for the purpose of nurturing one's own or another's spiritual growth."[3] Certainly, love involves exhilarating and tumultuous emotions, but these authors are referring to the work of love, the act of loving, what love looks like and how love behaves. This is love that can be encouraged and practiced. It is love that heals both lover and loved. And because this quality of love is the act of offering one's best self, in the Judeo-Christian tradition, it is commanded.

Adult love involves effort, commitment, and sacrifice. It is the task of safeguarding and nurturing the well-being of another. Love is complex and confusing because while it is joyful and fulfilling, it also requires the difficult task of managing the paradox of balancing love for another with love for oneself. Achieving that balance is the central and most difficult work in all loving relationships. It is the work of negotiating both gain and loss, of suffering and joy. And that task requires one of the most confusingly complex and difficult undertakings in any intimate interpersonal relationship, the task of negotiating perceptions. It is to that task we now turn.

Negotiating Perceptions

"Whose reality gets to be reality?" is one of the core conflicts in marriage. That conflict, underlying virtually all other conflict, is rarely addressed consciously, much less resolved. As I listen to couples argue from hour to hour, it's clear that underneath the surface conflict is an ongoing competition for who gets to be heard, who gets to be right, and which person's perception is "correct." People's perceptions differ about what happened, who's at fault, what was intended, what resulted, and who is crazy to think or feel the way they do. A lethal assumption in

---

3   Peck, S. (1978). *The Road Less Traveled*, p. 81.

relationships is that people need to agree on perceptions in order to solve problems or feel close. Even if, intellectually, a couple acknowledges that it's okay to agree to disagree, it is still emotionally challenging. We are afraid that if our significant other doesn't agree with our perceptions, they may misinterpret our actions, misunderstand our needs, mischaracterize our intentions, and misrepresent our thoughts and feelings. In other words, we're afraid they won't truly know us or genuinely accept us. Worse yet, we're afraid that, because of their own needs, they might not truly want to know us. If they did, they could feel responsible for how they treat us. And here is another tragic irony—our significant other typically feels the same way we do.

There are certainly parts of my personality that my spouse sees better than I do. I have reasons for not wanting to see those parts. I don't like them. They are parts of me that are selfish and inconsiderate. I would like to be a better person than I am. I would like to be a better husband, father, friend, therapist, and teacher, just to name a few of my roles. I would like to believe that I could be. It's hard for me to look at evidence that at times I'm not the person I would like to be. But I have a choice. I'll cite Scott Peck again. One of the disciplines of mature adulthood, of staying on the road less traveled, is one's commitment to the truth. The truth is that my spouse often sees me more clearly than I see myself. So I have a choice. What do I do with that truth?

Truth and Motive

Before I tackle that question, it's important to reflect on the possibility that there are parts of my spouse that I may see better than she does. I say "possibility" partly for political reasons and partly to make the point that I don't know for sure if I'm seeing the person that she truly is or the person that she is when she's with me, the person that I need her to be, the person that I project onto her, or the person I experience through the matrix of my previous experiences and emotional memories. Who is she really?

So now I have a real problem. I'm not sure that I truly know either one of us; and, in reality, that's a very good problem to have. It isn't an easy problem, just a very good one. If I can accept this *not knowing*, it may open up the possibility of new discoveries. If we are able to suspend our egos, our fears, and our need to be right, we just might be able to see things in ourselves that we haven't seen and perhaps haven't wanted to see. And here is the dividing line between a growing and stagnant relationship. When it comes to the test of whose reality gets to be reality, we have two choices. We can be *curious* or *competitive*. I can stubbornly cling to my own perceptions or be open to hers. I may not want to acknowledge this but in very real ways I need my spouse as a "reality consultant." And, hopefully, she is curious about my reality as well (come to think of it, she does think I'm a bit of a curiosity). If we can commit to staying open to each other and to each other's perceptions, we stand a much better chance of benefiting from each other's strengths, managing life more successfully, being much closer friends, and having a truly good marriage. We will help each other grow as individuals, support and encourage each other's gifts, and continue to discover more about ourselves and the love we share.

I once recommended to a husband, whose wife was much more focused and conscientious about their finances than he was, that rather than feel chronically guilty and irritated, he could appreciate that he had "hired" her (so to speak) as a consultant in areas where he was not as focused or motivated. It would, thus, be easier to let go of his competitiveness and value her strengths. She, in turn, was willing to see him as her consultant in acquiring more playfulness and balance. It worked. People can get too unnecessarily competitive and work too hard to "earn" love by trying to be omniscient or omni-competent. It doesn't work. It makes more sense to appreciate and applaud our spouse's strengths, and to feel good about the fact that we have strengths too.

I realize that I may be frustrating the reader at this point. Am I making too big a deal about perceptions and motivations and the requirements of true love? Isn't loving someone supposed to be easier? The answer is that it depends on your definition of love. It isn't hard to have loving feelings for someone, especially when those feelings are returned. It isn't hard to love how wonderful someone makes us feel. It isn't hard to exclaim love in the throes of passion. But, as I emphasized above, real love is hard work. It requires honest self-reflection, evaluating motives and behaviors, courageous vulnerability and trust, a willingness to negotiate needs and perceptions, and a daily commitment to the well-being of an *other*. Yes, genuine love is hard work, but it's worth it. The love that can happen between human beings is amazingly powerful. Truth and grace blended and embodied in love and offered from one person to another create the context in which one can experience healing and wholeness. To fully realize these possibilities, we turn next to the practical steps and essential skills of genuinely loving each other.

An important first step in that process is to have a good understanding of the role that emotions play in relationships. Artists, writers, film-makers, and musicians all know that emotion drives the story. But emotion isn't limited to telling creative stories; it extends to all stories. Even ethical thinking, according to Harvey Cox,[4] is driven by emotionally impactful stories. And because, like it or not, emotions usually decide whether a relationship is better or worse, I plan to take more time and go into more detail in the chapters on understanding and expressing emotions. First, we'll review the essential purpose and nature of emotions. Afterwards we will explore the topic of emotional honesty and the challenge of considering what or what not to bring up in your relationship. Then we'll look at psychological defenses: how they can get in the way and how to manage them. Finally, we will arrive at the central tasks of your work in couple therapy: helping your clients to become better friends, relate to each other more successfully, negotiate differences more skillfully, and, very possibly, love each other more deeply. For students, therapists, and others interested in a more academic discussion of emotions I recommend the following texts:

Chodorow, N. (1999). *The Power of Feeling.*
Damasio, A. (1994). *Descartes' Error: Emotion, Reason, and the Human Brain.*
Damasio, A. (1999). *The Feeling of What Happens: Body and Emotion in the Making of Consciousness.*
Damasio, A. (2003). *Looking for Spinoza: Joy, Sorrow, and the Feeling Brain.*
Ekman, P. (2003). *Emotions Revealed.*
Evans, D. (2001). *Emotion: The Science of Sentiment.*
Goleman, D. (1995). *Emotional Intelligence.*
Rolls, E. (2007). *Emotions Explained.*

---

4   Cox, H. (2006). *When Jesus Came to Harvard.*

Questions for Discussion

1. What are some of the qualities of your temperament that you like?
2. What are some of the qualities of your temperament that you dislike?
3. What might be qualities of temperament in a mate that would be attractive you?
4. In what ways would you like to become a more loving person?
5. What, from film or literature, exemplifies a loving person?
6. What, from film or literature, illustrates a person having to make a difficult but loving decision?

CHAPTER SIX

The Story of Emotion, Part 1

Understanding

CHAPTER SUMMARY AND LEARNING OBJECTIVE

In this chapter, I suggest a model for understanding the vital role that emotions play in survival and well-being. Even before the film *Inside Out* people have related emotions to various colors. People "see red" when they're angry, "feel blue" when depressed, and, for some reason, people (especially in Western movies) were called "yellow" when they were fearful. People "turn green" with envy, and so forth. The model I've suggested is very simple and easy to teach to clients. Emotions have a positive and negative polarity. The red of anger can also be the red of passion. Blue can be sad or serene. Yellow can be the scary dark of fear or the brilliant color of joy. The model is not just an easy way to understand emotion but also an important reminder that no "negative" emotion can be repressed without taking a toll on its positive complement. Repressing anger, for example, will result in numbing passion. Avoiding the blue of sadness will impede the essential grief process leading to acceptance and the blue of serenity and peace. The chapter also illuminates Antonio Damasio's description of three levels of emotion: primary, secondary, and background emotion. I conclude the chapter with a discussion of the existential concept of *angst*, the universal challenge of dealing with the inevitably of death and living in the tension between possibility and necessity.

> The learning objective for this chapter is to acquire confidence in presenting a model for explaining the role emotions play in relationships and the means to manage difficult emotion.

Primary Emotions

Virtually all therapy is concerned with emotion. It's important to understand the central role emotion plays in therapy. Simply put, emotions energize the work of survival. Survival for human beings and other mammals requires the instincts for both protection and connection. Emotions are in the service of both. Emotions such as fear and anger alert us to danger and energize us for self-protection. Emotions such as happiness and love signal sources of pleasure and secure attachments, other vital requirements for human survival.

Many researchers agree that human beings are born with what have been called *primary* or *basic* emotions. These are the emotions of happiness, sadness, fear, anger, shock or surprise, and disgust. Paul Ekhard, in his book *Emotions Revealed* (2003), describes the research he has done since the mid-1960s on how people recognize and experience emotions. Like many researchers in sociology, anthropology, and psychology, Ekhard originally believed that all emotions were learned and experienced differently from one people group to another. He was in the process of attempting to verify this belief when he discovered that his research was proving him wrong. Ekhard found that some emotions and their accompanying facial expressions are recognized and experienced similarly by all cultures around the globe. His photographs of the facial expressions of indigenous people of New Guinea and of similar expressions of emotions by Americans has been reproduced in many recent texts. Dylan Evans (2001), citing Ekhard's work, refers to the emotions listed above as "basic emotions." Anthony Damasio (2003) refers to the same list as "primary emotions." These are emotions that are instinctive rather than learned. They are the first emotions that human beings experience and express and they are the most important emotions for survival. In each sense, they are, indeed, primary. The function of these emotions is to provide the energy and incentive necessary to promote and protect one's own well-being and the well-being of one's significant attachments.

Happiness, for example, is a source of pleasure and the stimulus to maintain contact with the person or context in which that pleasure occurs. *Fear* is the energy that alerts us to danger and prompts us to create safety and protection from harm. *Anger* is the energy to create change; to confront a threat; to deal with a problem, person, or situation; and to establish and maintain boundaries. *Sadness* is the energy to let go of something or someone, to grieve the loss of an attachment, to arrive at a place of acceptance, and to repair oneself from loss. A startle response and the emotion of disgust put one on the alert that something could be dangerous or noxious. By being startled or disgusted, one is motivated to pay attention or to back away.

To reiterate, emotions are for *protection and connection*. That is to say, emotions are biochemical effects in our mind and body which protect us by warning us of danger, preparing us for fight or flight, arousing our passion or excitement, stirring us to appreciation and love, or calming us into a sense of contentment and well-being. We experience emotions on a continuum from intense pleasure to intense pain, rage, or terror. Emotions can be very complex and difficult to understand and express, but they are all important and necessary. People often want to pretend that they don't feel as they do, or they want to experience and express just the "positive" emotions and not the "negative"[1] ones. As a matter of fact, culture, not biology, has placed these values on emotions. All emotions are essentially *positive* in that they are important for survival. It is the *choices* that one makes in dealing with these emotions that can be positive or negative.

I'd like to suggest a useful way to think about emotions. Day after day, I sit with people who have difficulty talking to each other. This is typically because they have trouble being vulnerable. That is, people in conflict are much more inclined

---

1   Emotions are value neutral. My use of the terms "positive" and "negative" is similar to the positive–negative polarity of electric current.

to accuse one another than to be open about their own fears and hurts. Obviously, whatever their initial conflict, it's now become intensified by accusations and defenses. Here again we see that *content* issues become harder to discuss because of a dysfunctional *process*. When a couple decides to see me for marital therapy it's usually because they are beyond frustration and have begun to feel hopeless about ever being able to really talk to each other again or work things out.

The concept of "vulnerability" can be difficult for people. It seems that many people don't quite grasp the meaning of the word. To some, being vulnerable means being weak, unable to stand up for yourself, and susceptible to being hurt. That isn't the type of vulnerability I'm talking about. Being vulnerable in a relationship is a *choice*. It's a choice to feel. Vulnerability is the choice to be aware of and experience your own emotions or the emotions of another. It often requires courage; because being vulnerable means suspending one's psychological defenses and facing the threat of self-awareness and possible suffering. Being vulnerable means letting yourself truly care about another, with all of the emotional challenges that go with it. The other side of the coin is that being vulnerable also means being more available to intensely wonderful emotions—to passion, awe, and depths of love and caring. It's vital for people who love each other to practice learning to be vulnerable. This requires willingness, awareness, and skill. Remember that we are talking about the *work* of love. People work at becoming skilled at learning a language, playing an instrument, cooking, doing creative work, making wise investments, and perfecting their golf swing. Why not become more skilled at loving? When a couple comes in for therapy hopefully the *willingness* is there. But alongside of willingness there also needs to be courage. Seeing a counselor takes courage. It takes courage to honestly face oneself and to be open about aspects of yourself that are embarrassing or uncomfortable.

Let's return to our discussion of the nature and function of emotions. I've developed a very simple model to help clients remember primary emotions. That may seem unnecessary, but you'd be surprised at how many clients have a very limited emotional vocabulary. People know when they're happy, angry, or upset, but they aren't especially practiced at describing or recognizing many other types of emotions. The reason it's good to be more skilled in recognizing and describing emotion is because emotion is the principal currency of any ongoing relationship.

And in marriage, emotion is more than currency; it's the air you breathe.

The Color of Emotion

We've already learned about the various *primary* emotions. Using colors is a good way to remember them. Here is an exercise that will help you to see what I mean. The exercise will require a bit of imagination. I will ask you to imagine that you are going to paint four paintings. But before closing your eyes, I invite you to pretend that you are upstairs in your imaginary studio. There are four large blank canvases in each corner of the room with a dozen pots of paint and a large brush in front of each canvas. Imagine picking up a brush and, using whatever colors you wish, painting abstract pictures of the feelings of anger, sadness, depression, and happiness. Use any colors you like and put the paint on the canvas any way you choose. The first painting is of anger. The second is of sadness, and so forth. Okay, you can close your eyes and begin.

It's very interesting and useful for me to see how clients paint feelings. Looking at how they portray their emotions can be a good way to see how they *feel about how they feel*. When I look at how various emotions are expressed, using watercolor or poster paint, for example, it's interesting to notice the colors they choose, the intensity, the lights and the darks, the size and location of the emotion on the page, the manner in which the paint is applied, what efforts there are to contain or not contain the emotion, and whatever else the painter is depicting consciously or unconsciously. In the same manner that one might attempt to interpret a dream, I spread out each of the paintings and carefully ask about each one. I'm curious about each of the choices made. I ask about the painter's associations to the colors, the images, etc., in order to form an impression of the painter's relationships to his or her own emotions. Invariably, the painter responds to the exercise with fascination, surprise, and sometimes great relief that someone can truly understand and relate to the emotions that are being expressed and felt. People are typically fascinated by their own unconscious processes, surprised that their inner life can be seen and known, and relieved by the realization that they are both typically human and wonderfully unique. Painting, sculpture, collages, journaling, poetry, and dream work are a few of the revealing ways an individual can discover creative windows to the complexity and richness within.

I have looked at hundreds of paintings over the years. They are important windows for me to see inside the emotional soul of another and powerful ways for others to feel *seen* by me. In that sense, I use artwork both diagnostically and therapeutically. In paintings, I've seen panic attacks, chronic pain, dark rages, suicidal despair, and, all too often, terrible aloneness. If the paintings function to give me insight and, sometimes, a warning about the intensity of my patient's suffering, they also serve the patient as a way to sooth the unbearable feelings of aloneness and isolation. I always invite patients to keep their paintings, and many do. I am also blessed to have been given many paintings over the years and frequently use them when I teach on the topic of emotions.

Looking at a large collection of patient paintings, I have been impressed by how frequently people use similar colors to depict emotions. It's also interesting to me that the English language employs phrases that illustrate these typical colors. People "see red" when they're angry, "feel blue" when they're sad, and for some reason cowards were called "yellow" in old Western movies. So I've employed these common phrases to suggest a model that may make the tasks of understanding and expressing emotions a bit easier. Remember the color wheel that we were taught back in grade school? The primary colors were those that were not made from any other colors but were themselves used to create all of the remaining colors on the color wheel. Those primary colors are red, yellow, and blue. So a useful way to remember primary emotions is to think of them as primary colors. I suggested, above, that emotions serve survival and the attachment needs of *protection* and *connection*. As such, emotions are essential sources of information and energy. Some emotions are more comfortable than others, but they are all essential. If we set aside the emotions of happiness, shock or surprise, and disgust for the purposes of this model we can remember the three primary unpleasant emotions of anger, fear, and sadness from the primary colors above. When I ask students or patients to either imagine or actually paint these emotions, it isn't surprising that they typically paint anger as red or orange, sometimes mixing in black. The painting of anger can be explosive or quiet, subdued or fill the page. Sadness is usually depicted in blues or purples and typically painted to look drippy and fluid. Paintings of fear are scary. The colors are often a drab sickly yellowish hue, browns, oranges, or grays. If you did the creative imagination exercise above, what did your paintings look like? What colors did you use and how did you portray the emotion on your canvas?

Obviously, everyone has his or her own unique way of experiencing and depicting emotions; and one's culture will influence that experience. You may have discovered that the colors you associated with certain feelings were similar or different from the model I'm suggesting, but many people will use the colors described above to depict these primary emotions:

Anger

Fear   **Sadness**

On the other hand (or on the positive side), blue can be a calming color such as a blue sky or a tranquil lake. Red is the passionate color of Valentines and Chinese weddings. A bright yellow sun conveys a sense of faith, confidence, and courage. Recall that emotions are for protection and connection. In this way, I often think of emotions as double-sided coins or as a positive–negative electrical current. I don't like calling any emotion "negative," since each is so essential; however, if one considers emotions as having a kind of positive–negative polarity, it is easier to understand the dangers of repressing any of your emotions.

People usually hate feeling depressed and frightened, and most people don't like being angry. Growing up, many people were encouraged to keep their feelings to themselves, not to feel sorry for themselves, and not to be complainers. This was reinforced in sections of the American culture that have historically admired the lure of the rugged individual and the stoic pioneer who faced countless hardships without a murmur. Growing up as a typical American boy, I watched lots of movies. I only remember one film in which John Wayne shed a single tear. He portrayed a retiring cavalry officer who had been given a gold watch by his troopers. As he read the engraved inscription inside the watch he self-consciously wiped away a tear and steeled himself for his brief remarks. That was my cultural model for manhood: emotional restriction and stoicism.

I'm very fortunate, however, in having other role models. My father was born in Italy. Like me, he prizes the United States as a country and culture that offers the greatest opportunities for individual self-determination of any nation on the globe. But Dad held on to a bit of his old-world habits, so that at the same time I was watching John Wayne movies, my father was offering another role model for manliness: vulnerability and genuine affection. Parents from cultures that do not overrate stoicism, and emotionally intelligent parents from any culture, will appreciate that emotional maturity requires both *expressiveness* as well as *containment*. The old advice about children being seen and not heard doesn't work. Children need to be taught to express how they feel. But they also need to learn when and how to express themselves appropriately.

A new generation has been born, and I'm watching many dads and moms make better parenting decisions than their own parents. But many people are still very emotionally immature, and therapists are dealing daily with the physical, psychological, and relational consequences. So I have plenty of business. In fact, the profession of marriage and family therapy has exploded in the past 40 years. Hundreds of new therapists are licensed annually to deal with the outdated and deplorable consequences to individuals and families of this cultural habit of emotional stoicism.

I stated above that if people are unwilling to learn and rehearse communication skills, they will not have the quality of relationship that is possible for them, and the key to good communication is the willingness to be vulnerable. The reason that therapy is often required for relationships is that people are typically unskilled at expressing feelings and too practiced at defending against the feelings of others. Effective therapists help people to get over the habit of repressing feelings and acquire the habit of non-defensive listening. Yes, these are difficult habits to learn, but completely worth it. This is because while repression is a hard habit to break, the cost of repressing our "negative" emotions is that we then lose access to our "positive" emotions. Emotions are emotions—we can't pick and choose. We must take the dark with the light. To feel fully alive, to feel both passion and peace, we can't run away from painful emotions. Our capacity for intense joy is determined by our willingness to acquire tolerance for pain.

I can't emphasize too strongly the importance of acquiring the skill and tolerance for accessing and expressing all emotions. Because emotions tend to be "double-sided," repressing anger is also repressing passion. People get angry about situations or people that they care about. Passion connects us to important people in our lives, and to important places and causes. That's why I don't get nervous when people in my office are angry at each other. In my mind, they still care. There's still some passion. I can work with that, and with them. What is really hard is trying to repair indifference. The opposite of love isn't anger; it's indifference.

There isn't very much a therapist can do when a wife says, "I simply don't care anymore. He can do whatever he wants to try to save this marriage and it won't do any good. I am done!" I will have a lot more to say about dealing with difficult emotions later. For the present, it's important for me to repeat that *passion* is the energy to connect. *Anger* is information about what isn't working and the energy to fix it. *Sadness* is the energy to grieve a loss, to let go of an attachment and to heal. Allowing yourself to grieve will eventually help you to let go, and acquire acceptance, peace, and *serenity*. Avoiding sadness or grief only leads to bitterness or chronic hostility—an inability to let go. This is why humility, vulnerability, and forgiveness are so important for mental health.

Fear is the energy to be alert to danger, to take precautions, or do something to prevent harm. Fear isn't pleasant but it is one of the most prominent of all human emotions. The opposite of fear is *confidence* or *courage*. I'm not sure whether confidence is an emotion or a mental state that positively affects emotions. I'm inclined to think that it is the latter. Clearly courage is a commitment to a course of action in spite of one's fears. Nonetheless, for the purpose of remembering that emotions are double-sided (protection/connection), I will include confidence as the connective side of the protective emotion of fear. Below is an expanded view of a useful model to remember our primary emotions. No doubt people have used colors to describe emotions for thousands of years, so it seems to be a convenient model for simplifying the task of remembering our most basic emotions.

Anger/Passion

Fear/Confidence   **Sadness/Serenity**

Notice the connection between sadness and serenity, two sides of the color blue. Likewise, there is the double-sided red of anger and of passion. There is the sickly, pale yellow of fear and the bright exuberant yellow of confidence. Human emotion can be very dynamic.

Emotions can quickly transition from one to another and from one intensity to another. To complicate matters, like hues on a color wheel, emotions can be combined to form new emotions. Anger, for example, when repressed by fear, can be transformed into the *emergency orange* of anxiety or condensed into black rage. When people paint pictures using both the red of anger and the blue of sadness they often include the color black, suggesting the feeling of being stuck. A lot of black in a painting can portray hopelessness or despair. People paint in purple and blue hues when they're sad. Depression, however, is often portrayed as a muting or washing out of all of the colors. Depressed people often describe themselves as not feeling much of anything or of being emotionally numb.

Emotions also have a way of hiding. Hurt and fear, for example, often hide under anger.

Anger as a stronger, more powerful emotion often exists on the surface, disguising and arising from the more vulnerable emotions underneath. A careful listener, however, may detect a frightened or hurting person behind an angry scolding or a cold withdrawal. Remember that emotions tell us about how we are experiencing an event. In some instances, emotions give us good information about what is really happening. At other times, an event may trigger old emotions which color our perception of what is really happening in the present. In any case, emotions are important sources of information and must be examined and understood. I have included a list of some common feeling words in the appendix. They are arranged with the darker hues on top and their lighter counterparts on the bottom. The lists are also arranged from lesser intensity hues on top to greater intensity hues on the bottom.

People sometimes ask where words like "confusion" or "happiness" or "joy" fit into the model. Confusion may exist when someone isn't sure which emotion he or she is feeling. Feeling a number of different emotions simultaneously can also be confusing. Sometimes confusion exists because of an inner conflict between the actual feeling and what one thinks is acceptable to feel. The emotion of happiness results from a *happening*. "This *experience* makes me happy," for example, "My children, spouse, or friends make me happy. I am happy with my life right now." Joy is a spiritual experience. It is a difficult-to-define sense of well-being that may exist even in the *midst* of difficulties. Joy may be a deep knowing that all is as it should be or an inexplicable awareness of God's presence.

Secondary Emotions

Secondary emotions are *social* emotions. They are learned in the social contexts of home and culture. Emotions such as envy, jealousy, guilt, shame, and embarrassment, as well as sympathy and pride, are acquired in specific ways and in specific contexts depending on cultural and family norms. Like primary emotions, secondary emotions can be both beneficial as well as troublesome. On the one hand, secondary or social emotions provide the emotional cues and incentives to help us maintain or enhance affiliation and attachment. On the other hand, once imprinted by cultural and family conditioning, these secondary emotions can be extremely intense and persistent in regulating and maintaining behavior in ways that are healthy and beneficial as well as in ways that are toxic and binding. A social emotion may be an extension of a primary emotion. Antonio Damasio[2] suggests that the emotion of contempt, for example, while considered a social emotion, has its roots in the primary emotion of disgust. The look of contempt is remarkably similar to the look of disgust. In that context, the word *disgusting* is used to refer to a person or situation that is able to invoke the social equivalent of something toxic.

Shame may be the most common social emotion. Clearly, shame is experienced and expressed differently in different cultures and families and elicits the emotional cohesion that rigidly regulates every aspect of family life. In certain families, shame is felt not just for behaving inappropriately but for behaving independently. In these families, a family member is not permitted to be an individual—to think, feel, or behave differently than the norms tolerated by family tradition. John Bradshaw describes this as toxic shame.[3]

OF APPETITES AND EMOTIONS

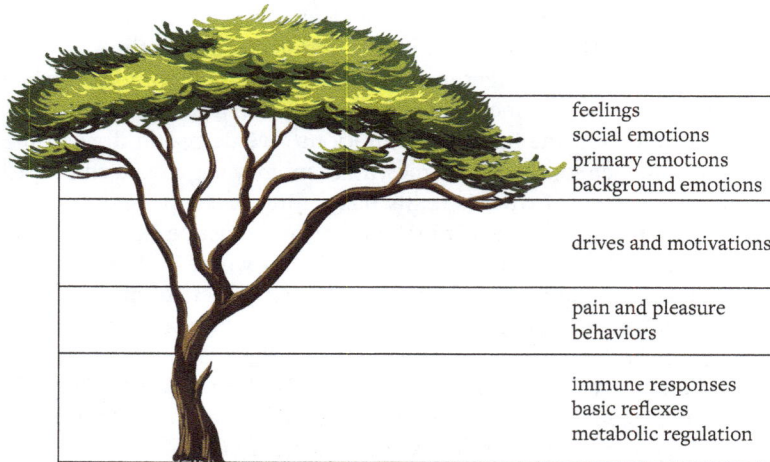

feelings
social emotions
primary emotions
background emotions

drives and motivations

pain and pleasure
behaviors

immune responses
basic reflexes
metabolic regulation

FIG. 6-1 There are at least three kinds of emotion-proper: background emotions, primary emotions, and social emotions. The nesting principle applies here, too. For example, social emotions incorporate responses that are part of primary and background emotions.

a) Source: Antonio R. Damasio, "Primay, Secondary, and Background Emotions," Looking for Spinoza. Copyright © 2003 by Harcourt Inc. b) Copyright © 2012 Depositphotos/Interactimages.

Bradshaw describes family systems in which a member feels shame for being him or herself. This type of toxic shame is one of the most common and, unfortunately, one of the most difficult emotions to heal. When shame has been internalized at a young age it does more than effectively regulate behavior, it kills a child's spirit. Shame insidiously permeates one's being and becomes woven into the psyche. Breathing the atmosphere in a toxic family can, over time, so expose one to shame and anxiety that one's body itself is affected. The net consequence is that a person carries the sometimes subtle, sometimes intense, feelings of shame deep within

2   Damasio, A. (2003). *Looking for Spinoza*, p. 45.
3   Bradshaw, J. (1988). *Healing the Shame that Binds You.*

his or her core Self. Persistent exposure to any conditioned emotional experience does, in fact, alter one's physiology. That conditioned, pervasive, affective-somatic interface is what Damasio[4] has called "background emotion." Many people have a background emotion of anxiety. They often find themselves feeling restless or jittery. Other background emotions may be depressive, or hostile, or, for some, lighthearted. These background emotions are so ingrained and familiar that we hardly notice the effect they have on our moods, our thoughts, and our physical health. They are truly "in the background." Below, a diagram from Damasio's *Looking for Spinoza* shows the relationship between primary, secondary, and background emotions.

In the diagram above, notice how the body's registration of pleasure and pain branches into a myriad of drives and motivations. These drives and motivations become habituated, over time, and affect the nature and degree of physical and emotional arousal, leading to a conditioned state of background emotion. Background emotions constitute a subtle emotional interface between the body and the surrounding environment. An individual is hardly ever conscious of this body state until it's lifted into awareness by circumstances or the act of disciplined attunement or mindfulness. For example, a person may not realize that he or she is anxious most of the time. People may tend to "run" anxious and not realize it until they make an effort to set aside habitual behaviors that absorb or mask anxiety. I often suggest to my clients that one way to gauge their level of background anxiety is to spend one minute after getting into their car before turning on the ignition; and then to spend one minute after turning off the ignition before reaching for the door handle. Try that exercise. It's a lot harder than you might imagine. Try doing it for three days in a row. You'll likely give up after the first day. It's that hard to break the habit of "running" anxious. While you're waiting for the endless sixty seconds to elapse, meditate, pray, think of things you are grateful for, or, even better, try not to think of anything at all. It's difficult to step out of the "blur" of incessant obligation, but it is a good discipline to work on.

Anxiety is probably one of the most common background emotions, but there are others. Some people seem depressed or melancholic most of the time. Others seem to be angry or chronically hostile. When asked, "Are you angry?" people with this background emotion are so accustomed to the emotion that they usually say no, not realizing that they are frequently sending unconscious messages that they are unhappy, irritated, or just don't want to be bothered. Angry body language is pretty hard to mistake.

Some fortunate individuals are genuinely happy and optimistic most of the time. Their predominant background emotion seems to be lighthearted and positive. It seems as if people do sort of "breathe in" the pervasive emotional climate in their environment growing up and that emotional climate is absorbed into their being. Their physiology habituates this pervasive emotional state and, with time, that emotional state becomes a consistent "background" emotion.

This is where I typically find myself wanting to argue with cognitive therapists who imagine that instructing people to think differently is all it takes to change how people feel. If I wanted to be ill-mannered, I would suggest that David Burns' book *Feeling Good* states, simplistically, "don't think that—think this" and all will be well. In defense of Burns, however, I have often recommend his books to folks who need to work hard at "don't think that—think this."

---

4   Damasio, A. (2003). *Looking for Spinoza.*

More often, I suggest they read Burns' *Feeling Good Workbook* and do the exercises Burns recommends. Burns is correct—if one could learn to govern one's thought life it would greatly benefit one's emotional life. Most depressive states, Burns correctly emphasizes, are caused by the habit of self-defeating thinking.

But my argument with Burns and other cognitive therapy purists is "good luck with that." For a person who grew up breathing in the environment of two depressed parents, for example, their brain and body have been so conditioned and imprinted with the background emotion of depression that it may require years of reconditioning neural pathways in order to undo the damage.

Background emotions do seem to be a more subtle, pervasive, and habituated extension of primary emotions. Much of the time people do experience quieter forms of fear, anger, sadness, or happiness in ways that are less intense and conscious. As a result, it doesn't take much to trigger a more intense experience of these same emotions. Paying attention to recurring emotional triggers is one of the best ways to learn more about these background emotional states and to make some progress in regulating or improving them.

It is much easier to become conscious of one's background emotional state than it is to alter it. Therapists are often bedeviled by clients who perfectly understand what is wrong with them and how they *ought* to think, feel, or behave—but don't. The major emphasis of cognitive-behavioral therapy is to help people see that their emotions and behaviors arise from negative, dysfunctional thoughts and habits. Clients are encouraged to recognize and confront these automatic thoughts and their underlying core beliefs and to substitute more rational, logical, and reality-based thinking. This is a very effective and, typically, a very useful form of therapy. Neophyte therapists, however, and people reading self-help books want to believe that changing one's habits of thinking, feeling, and behaving is much easier than it truly is. Dieting and exercising regularly, for example, are great ideas, but easier said than done, especially if a person is up against the resistance of unconscious emotions and conflicted motivations.

A psychodynamic approach to therapy works better for getting to the root of hidden emotions and unconscious conflicts. Modern psychodynamic therapy has evolved to include an appreciation for the significance of early attachments and the role that childhood conditioning and emotional imprinting plays in the emotional development of the infant.

Research has shown how the brain develops in relationship to significant others in the formative years, and how both brain and body respond to these positive and negative emotional influences. Dan Siegel's *The Developing Mind* (1999) and Louis Cozolino's *The Neuroscience of Human Relationships* (2006) are must-reads in the area of early childhood attachment patterns and their relationship to brain development. Effective therapy involves more than helping people change dysfunctional habits of thinking, feeling, and behaving. For therapy to be truly effective it is important to recognize that biochemistry itself needs to be transformed. For that reason, it is important to understand the nature and function of the habituated physiological state of background emotions and their role in how we feel and behave.

Angst

Angst, as a philosophical term, describes the human condition of living daily with some level of awareness that one will eventually die. Human beings are conscious that they are finite. They may choose not to think about that fact, but the fact will not go away. Each human being is unique, valuable, and potentially very creative. Human beings frequently believe that their life has meaning, that they matter, that they have something to give or leave behind for the next generation. It is painful to consider that life is short and may end without one's having lived a truly meaningful life. The word used for this type of pain is *angst*, the unavoidable "background emotion" of being human. Physical and emotional symptoms originate not only from toxic relationships, but also from this pervasive and deep-seated type of anxiety.

I often wonder, in a marriage ceremony, do couples understand that among the things they are promising to negotiate with each other is suffering? Our attraction to marriage is, in part, our desire to be happy. At a deeper, unconscious level, our attraction to marriage is an attraction to growth, to becoming a larger person. There is tremendous potential in a good relationship to learn to live fully—to experience genuine acceptance, grace, and wholeness. But one cannot be open to those experiences without also being open to the unavoidable realities of suffering, pain, and loss.

Ideally, love is learned early in the family, practiced in one's relationships, exercised and perfected over time to energize the work of making a difference in the world. But that ideal is shared by too few people. They lack the courage. A much safer goal for many is to simply get by. A significant symptom of modern living is the need to be "normal," to be satisfied with a house in the suburbs, a two-week vacation, and a retirement on the golf course. Too often the need to be *normal* is realized by one's becoming *invisible* by fitting in, not standing out, satiated by the mundane—in the words of Soren Kierkegaard, "tranquilized in trivia."[5] According to existential psychology, the need to be liked, and to be like everybody else, is the most pervasive disorder of our time.

Therapists attempt to help people find ways to resolve problems and have happier marriages and relationships. That is a good and valuable thing to do. But there are greater goals in life than these. A greater goal is to become a person who is competent in loving, and with love, to help the ones loved to reach their potential. The ultimate function of marriage is to extend grace and strength to another human being, to face all the pain and fear of being human, and to work together to bring something of value into the world.

> *And your arms felt nice wrapped 'round my shoulders—And I had a feeling that I belonged—I had a feeling I could be someone, be someone, be someone.*

"Fast Car," Tracy Chapman

It's good to understand these many different types of emotions, their functions, and effects because they constitute the currency of relationships. But understanding emotions is much easier than managing them. As with other forms of currency, mishandling one's emotions can be devastating. So we turn now to the multifaceted task of learning to manage emotions. And the first of these tasks is to learn how to express them.

---

5 Kierkegaard, S. (1894). *The Sickness Unto Death*, p. 174–175.

Questions for Discussion

1. What colors did you use in the painting exercise? Did any of the colors you chose surprise you?
2. How did you place the paint on the paper to describe a particular emotion or context?
3. What did you learn from the painting exercise?
4. What other types of creative processes might you use with clients to express their emotions?
5. What do you think may be your main background emotion(s)?
6. How and in what context are you able to experience background emotions?
7. Have you had times in your life when you were aware of a sense of angst?
8. Do you recall what, if anything, you did in response to experiencing angst?

CHAPTER SEVEN

The Story of Emotion, Part 2

Expressing

CHAPTER SUMMARY AND LEARNING OBJECTIVE

This chapter deals with the challenge of being honest with one's feelings. It's one thing to understand emotions; it's another to effectively manage them. This is especially true in uncomfortable conversations. Our fight/flight defenses get in the way. Whether attacking or avoiding, emotions can drive perceptions, and people find themselves wrestling with distorted thoughts and inflamed or buried emotions. Deborah Tannen has researched different communication styles in males and females. Temperament and family conditioning also play a large role in informing styles of communication. All of us can benefit from learning and practicing the skills necessary to suspend defenses, be emotionally honest as the speaker, and open and non-defensive as the listener.

The learning objective for this chapter is to be confident in describing the essential role of psychological defenses and the importance of developing skills and strategies to manage them.

Emotional Honesty

We learn from our parents and from our culture which emotions are acceptable to express, and even which emotions are acceptable to feel. We learn how and when and to whom to express our emotions. And, for many of us, what we've learned has caused us some pretty serious problems. Have I said that all emotions are important and necessary? The reason I keep repeating myself is because day after day I try to help people undo the consequences of bad emotional training. Serious problems exist when people are unable to access or express emotions. Emotions that go unrecognized and unexpressed can develop a life of their own. Held captive in the unconscious, the three prisoners—anger, fear, and sadness—look for avenues of escape. They escape into the body with physical symptoms, into the mind with dark moods and depression, and into relationships with anxious thoughts, angry outbursts, and unresolved tensions.

Many years ago, there was an unfortunate trend in the "encounter movement" encouraging followers to uncritically vent all emotion, regardless of the context. The idea behind this teaching was intended to be a corrective to the very emotionally repressive habits of earlier decades. While emotional honesty is important for mental health it is not the *prime* ethic. Yes, it could be argued that more damage comes from the consequences of repressing emotions than from responsibly expressing them. But emotional honesty is not the supreme value. Honesty must always be in the service of love.

I agree with M. Scott Peck in *The Road Less Traveled*, that although commitment to the truth or "dedication to reality," as Peck refers to it, is essential for individual and relational well-being, there are times when it is more loving to keep quiet. Peck suggests some guidelines for when it might be more loving to make the difficult decision to keep your feelings and opinions to yourself. I encourage individuals, couples, and families to review his suggestions in *The Road Less Traveled*. Peck believes in open and honest relationships and the importance of challenging oneself to be authentic. Consequently, evaluating one's motives for either disclosing or withholding emotional honesty requires careful self-examination. The fruit of that frequent in-depth and loving reflection is spiritual growth.

Reading Scott Peck's advice for the first time was both reassuring and personally refreshing. I have an illustration. Some time ago, without any conversation or negotiation, my wife and I made a deal to periodically lie to each other. It's an interesting sort of lie, because the purpose of the lie is to be able to tell the truth. When she and I are out to dinner and a very attractive woman walks by behind her, I make a conscious effort to disobey my biology and avoid staring. I suppose that might be a form of emotional dishonesty, but my biology isn't the final truth. The truest truth is that, for me, there is no one more beautiful or amazing than my wife. It is that truth that I choose to affirm. Conversely, I know that I'm not the most attractive or interesting man around, but I don't know that from my wife. A truth, at one level, is that I'm not especially unique or interesting or important. But because of her love, I get to feel that way.

Which is the truer truth? Of course, I'm well aware that if Sean Connery were walking behind me in a restaurant, the deal would be off. I guess it's important for me to remember *that* truth as well

Knowing what "truths" to share and how and when to share them, and in what contexts to exercise discretion, requires the motivation of love and the discipline of maturity. As I mentioned previously, one of the most interesting and challenging tasks of a relationship is to negotiate reality. I listen to a dozen or so marital arguments each week. A central debate in each of these arguments is whose reality gets to be the reality. But the debate is less about perceptions than about emotions. Partners are afraid of differences. They assume that they need to agree about perceptions in order to have meaningful conversations, solve problems, or feel close. They argue that if they can't agree on a common reality, how can they resolve differences or make correct decisions? People spend a great deal of time and emotion trying to prove their point of view, their recollection of an event, their solution to the problem, or that the other person is wrong. This is not only painful and a waste of time, but it also undermines the openness and trust essential for working toward solutions.

I frequently listen to people appeal to their partner for emotional honesty. Often, this is a legitimate appeal. Ideally, if an emotion is felt strongly and often, it ought to voiced. But there are two difficulties with the concept of emotional honesty. One difficulty is that the appeal for honesty is frequently used to hurt or control people: "I'm just being honest," they say. "I'm telling you this for your own good—if I didn't love you …" and so forth. These are frequently preambles to insensitive, hurtful, and sometimes manipulative ways of getting the upper hand in a relationship. The second difficulty is with the concept of emotional honesty itself. Emotions are not necessarily honest.

Sometimes I ask myself whether one emotional experience is truer than another, or if either emotion is "true" in the sense that the emotion truly corresponds to anything that is happening to me right now. Am I being visited by an emotional "Ghost of Christmas Past"—haunted by emotions I felt when I was eight years old? In these situations, my brain is indifferent to what year it is. What my brain knows is that this present situation resembles the experience that I had when I was eight. As a result, what I felt *then* could be overlaid on what I'm feeling *now*. So is it a "true" feeling? It feels true. But here's the tricky part. At the same time I'm feeling this present emotion, I'm also feeling, uncomfortably, like an eight-year-old. I don't much like feeling like an eight-year-old. So now I have an emotion about an emotion. What does that do to my original emotion? And what about the background emotion that I had as an eight-year-old, is that present as well? How much "truth" can I really gather from all of this, and how much of this truth is *true* enough to disclose with any real or useful implications for my relationship?

So, while I do like the idea of emotional honesty, I'm not sure how honest my emotions are. Among the most interesting and therapeutic conversations in my marriage have to do with exploring (with someone who truly loves me, trusts me, and is patient with me) what the heck is going on with me emotionally. But as much as I enjoy and value those conversations, they also scare me. I wonder, at times, if I'm being too vulnerable. Is being "real" really a good idea? How much of me does my wife genuinely want to know. Even though she's a therapist, she's not *my* therapist and my guess is that there are probably things better left unsaid.

It's valuable to consider what is important and necessary to bring up in the realm of emotional honesty. There is value in considering which feelings are relevant to today and important to disclose and which are not. Sometimes I decide that what I'm feeling is my own responsibility to deal with and I don't need to bother my wife about it. The problem, for me, is that I'm tempted to decide that too often. Like many males, I shy away from emotional conflict, I often don't trust my feelings, and I tend to feel shame when I feel needy or vulnerable, so I typically keep my feelings to myself. Or at least that's what I would like to think. But then I remind myself of the communication rule I stated above: one cannot *not* communicate. I can communicate directly and responsibly or indirectly with a bad mood, irritability, or emotional distance. I now know that when there is a problem in my relationship and I have some uncomfortable feelings about it, whether I like it or not, those feelings will be communicated one way or another. It's my choice.

I do think about whether my feelings are important enough to share with my spouse or whomever. And I do think about the best way to bring them up. And, as I've said, it's easier for me not to bring them up, so I usually push myself to do it. But for many people the opposite is true. There are probably just as many people who need to practice *containment* as those who need to practice *expressiveness*. It frequently seems to me that half of the population coming to see me for therapy needs to practice opening up and the other half needs to practice clamming up.

Maybe this is because the "flight" defense is easier for some and the "fight" defense is easier for others. It reminds me of what Harville Hendrix said about "fusers" and "isolators," above.

In my experience, some people do seem to have a greater need for the felt sense of emotional connection and others do not. I've wondered, over the years, why these two types of people are very often attracted to each other and marry. And that's when things certainly become more interesting.

Some people might immediately identify with the idea of needing to *fuse* or *isolate*. For others, the terms *demonstrative* and *independent* are more accurate and less pejorative. What Hendrix is pointing out is that people who use these two different defensive strategies to manage the dynamics of closeness and independence not only tend to be attracted to each other but their relationship can easily drift into what has been termed a *regressive cycle*. A regressive cycle occurs when each person's defensive style tends to push the other into a more entrenched defensive position—a reaction, in other words, to the others reaction. I think most therapists would agree with Hendrix's observation regarding the existence of regressive cycles in relationships. I think that they would also agree with how very difficult it is to turn those cycles around.

For the *isolator*, the challenge is to be open and vulnerable, to care about the other enough to risk expressing painful and potentially explosive feelings. For the *fuser* it means not assuming that every negative thought or emotion is the other partner's responsibility to fix, and to learn how to be more disciplined and skillful in what, when, and how to express oneself.

And for both, it means learning how to work together to develop the strategies and guidelines necessary to create enough safety and trust to learn from each other. It is to that end that I developed the communication guidelines I've included in the appendix. They are very simple guidelines. They need to be simple for reasons I will explain. But even though the guidelines are simple, they are not easy.

Hopefully, as a therapist, you will spend much of your time helping your couple to practice skills. Clearly, in the initial phase of therapy your focus will be on getting information, agreeing on goals for therapy, and developing trust. The couple may be in crisis and need to get some help with creating stability and deciding on a direction. After the crisis eases and your couple is in a better place emotionally, you will want to help them to learn and practice skills. The focus of therapy will shift from lecture to lab. Since little help is gained by insight alone, you'll need to make sure they can learn to talk to each other successfully without your help. Your goal is to become redundant.

I can watch my golf instructor and listen to his suggestions, but very soon I'll have to grip the club myself. It may be that because classic psychoanalysis relied too heavily on "interpretation," behavioral therapy was developed as an essential corrective. So, while insight is valuable and it's good to have (you, the therapist, provide some traffic control and peacekeeping in the initial sessions of therapy), it's critical that most of your therapy be spent doing the "lab work" of rehearsing skills. Your clients have to go home after the session, and they'll need the skills to do their own peacekeeping. Like a golf swing, those skills will have to be rehearsed again and again so that they'll be accessible in the presence of heated emotions. That's why the guidelines I've included in the appendix, while easy to understand, are difficult to apply and require lots of practice.

I shouldn't leave this chapter without explaining why many males have difficulty expressing emotion at times. John Gray[1] suggested that the difficulty had to do with anatomy—the fact of being male; and because males are so emotionally stunted, they must be from Mars. I didn't find a great deal of research supporting Gray's conclusions. I did find a great deal of entertainment value.

A more persuasive insight into male communication style comes from Deborah Tannen's research.[2] As a sociolinguist, Tannen noticed how male children are often socialized differently than female children. In Tannen's words, males are allowed, in some cases even encouraged, to be more competitive, while females are socialized to be more cooperative. I think Tannen is right about this. I frequently ask the males in my classes to recall their experience as youngsters, especially when they were in junior high or middle school. Virtually all of the males report that they would have felt ashamed to talk about vulnerable emotions with other males. They would expect to be called a bad name and ridiculed. Most of the girls in the class report a very different experience. They recall feeling permission to be vulnerable with their female friends. They would usually anticipate and experience comforting and would subsequently learn how to give comfort. I have heard many wives express disappointment that their male partners were reluctant to be vulnerable and didn't know how to be comforting. Most males tell me that they are uncomfortable with vulnerability and, in fact, often feel ashamed to express it. So it does seem that socialization has a great deal to do with how comfortable males and females are with expressing emotion. It's also clear why most therapists expect to encounter challenges in their couple counseling when wives report being disappointed that their husbands aren't emotionally accessible or expressive. And husbands, in turn, complain that talking about feelings is not something they're comfortable with. But more satisfying than simply appealing to the idea that men are from Mars, it would be good for males, unpracticed at expressing vulnerable emotions, to learn how.

This is where you come in. After exploring the communication pattern of your couple, you'll want to point out what you see. You'll remind your couple that all relationships are unique, and yet there are familiar patterns from one relationship to the next. In some cases, it's the male who is the more expressive, and in some cases the female. In some cases, neither is very expressive (although that's pretty rare). In some cases, both partners are very expressive—like our middle daughter and her Italian husband. I'm guessing that my tendency to see one partner as more expressive in a relationship, and the other less, is a function of the prevailing culture around me.

Questions for Discussion

1. What do you think—how do you remember your parents' communication style?
2. Using Hendrix's terms, do you think you are more of a fuser or isolator?
3. In what contexts would it be better to "withhold truth"?
4. Growing up, what messages do you recall about expressing emotions?

1 Gray, J. (1992). *Men Are from Mars, Women Are from Venus*.
2 Tannen, D. (2007). *You Just Don't Understand: Women and Men in Conversation*.

CHAPTER EIGHT

The Story of Communication

CHAPTER SUMMARY AND LEARNING OBJECTIVE

This chapter outlines the skills required for successful communication between couples. In their textbook on family therapy, Goldenberg and Goldenberg state that "all behavior is communication at some level." They are saying that people cannot *not* communicate. Whether overtly or covertly, emotions will express themselves. Depression, hostility, distancing, sniping are examples of dishonest communication. Bad communication habits are hard to break. A good therapist will do more than simply point out what couples are doing wrong. He or she will teach them skills, and, like a good trainer, will make sure that couples develop emotional strengths and skills to communicate successfully. Insight is valuable in therapy; even more valuable is practice. The Parent, Adult, Child model developed by Eric Berne is a very useful metaphor to help people gain insight into the origin of both inner and outer conflicts. The communication rules and exercises I've outlined in the appendix provide the training regimen that couples can rehearse to build essential relationship strengths.

The learning objective for this chapter is the ability to apply skills and strategies essential for successful communication, the core competency, in relationships.

Confusing Messages

There are two hurdles we need to get over if we want to communicate successfully. The first hurdle has to do with how we listen and what we hear. Everyone has had the experience of not feeling understood or feeling misunderstood. It can feel pretty crazy and frustrating when we try hard to get our message across and another person isn't "getting it" or doesn't want to get it. That brings up the second hurdle, defensiveness. Who hasn't said or heard the words "don't be so defensive!" That's easier said than done. I'll spend some time discussing why we get defensive and how to better manage our defenses. But first we need to look at the challenge of getting one's message across.

Communication can be difficult and confusing because of the complexity of spoken and unspoken messages involved. There is, at a minimum, the message the speaker intends to send and the message the listener hears. Happily, these two messages may be close enough in meaning to successfully convey the information. Even so, we have all become accustomed to snags in communication. A good book to read on this topic is Deborah Tannen's *That's Not What I Meant!*[1] Tannen does a great job of clarifying why messages can be so easily misunderstood. She examines the difference between the *intent* of the message and its *effect* on the listener (I think there is always some difference). Tannen also explains why people frequently respond more to how a message is delivered or "packaged" than to the content of the message itself.

When it comes to emotions, the task of sending and receiving information is especially complex. Emotions are very individual and unique. They develop from millions of conditioned cues people learn growing up. They are also conditioned by experiences and emotional injuries later in life. Our emotional responses are also very subjective. It's a wonder that anyone can successfully communicate at all. Probably the most complicated emotion to express and experience is love. What is the speaker saying when he or she says, "I love you," and what does the listener hear? What expectations result? Virtually all the emotional work in a romantic relationship revolves around the many messages surrounding the meaning of the word love.

Another serious hindrance to clear communication, besides the different meanings we attach to words, is the way in which the message is conveyed, the tone of voice, the inflection, the body language, and so forth. Linguists call this the *meta-message*. The meta-message is the *unspoken* message that influences the content of what we are saying. How often have you heard, "It's not what you said—it's the way you said it"? The meta-message is how meaning is packaged. And the packaging of a message can change its meaning—how one says what one says can make the listener amused, confused, or furious. The meta-message is how we feel about what we say and what expectations we have about how we want our listener to respond.

Goldenberg and Goldenberg, in their textbook on family therapy, have this to say about meta-messages and the effects on the narrative systems in relationships:

- All behavior is communication at some level.
- Communication may occur simultaneously at many levels—gestures, body language, tone of voice, posture, intensity—in addition to the content of what is said.
- Every communication has content (report) and a relationship (command) aspect. (By the word "command," the authors are referring to the speaker's expectations of how the message should be perceived.)
- Each person punctuates a sequence of events in which he or she is engaged in different ways. Problems develop and are maintained within the context of interactive patterns and feedback loops.[2]

The *unspoken* message or meta-message is often heard as the *real* message because it can indicate how someone *really* feels. On the other hand, the listener

---

1   Tannen, D. (2011). *That's Not What I Meant*.
2   Goldenberg, H., & Goldenberg, I. (2004). *Family Therapy*, p. 243–245.

may be just as likely to read into the other's body language or tone of voice his or her own subjective interpretation or emotional response to what is being said. This is what therapists refer to as *transference*.

Transference is experiencing another person from within the matrix of one's own previous emotional conditioning. In other words, in transference, you really aren't experiencing the other person at all. You are not experiencing them as *other*. You are experiencing more of your own subjective emotional reaction to the other.

In intersubjective systems theory Robert Stolorow emphasizes the importance of therapists being fully aware of the transference and countertransference dynamics at play in therapy. Although cognitive and emotional biases exist largely in the unconscious, those dynamics are co-constellated between therapist and client and impact the process of therapy.

It is not possible, according to Stolorow, for a therapist to imagine that he or she is able to hold an authoritative, God's-eye view of pathology. With a view to postmodern thought, the observer cannot be separated from that which is being observed.

While it is true that all of our experiences are our own subjective emotional reactions and there is no such thing as unbiased perception, there is a great deal of difference between a tentative and curious *response* to one's perceptions and an arrogant, self-convinced *reaction* that is loaded with defensive anger or anxiety. Our emotional reactions to people and the consequent distortions of meaning constitute our psychological defenses. Obviously, there are times when it is appropriate to feel angry or anxious, as well as sad or depressed. But it is also important to acquire the discipline of curiosity and mature reflection in order to wisely respond to these emotions. A good definition of a mature relationship is that partners characteristically *respond* to each other instead of merely *reacting*.

Anyone can react. Reactions do not require training, wisdom, or love. They do not involve or promote maturity. Responses do. Responses require the *discipline of choice*, and choice, in tense situations, requires practice. Your couple needs to practice *responding* to each other instead of *reacting*. This will require their practicing taking time to identify their emotions and stepping back, briefly, to analyze the situation before responding. In this process, some people will learn to take a deep breath, perhaps pray for guidance or wisdom, or simply consider the best option for a response. Recall the old prayer:

> *God grant me the serenity to accept the things I cannot change; courage to change the things I can; and wisdom to know the difference.*
>
> Reinhold Niebuhr

With motivation and practice, one can respond to others in ways that are wise and even loving. This is one of the steps in acquiring what Goleman termed "emotional intelligence."[3] Before we can go further in describing the skills necessary to respond to people instead of react to them, it's important to become more familiar with some of our typical psychological defenses.

---

3   Goleman, D. (2005). *Emotional Intelligence.*

Dealing with Defenses

The most profound and pervasive human emotion is fear. We fear for our physical safety and well-being, and when we're not preoccupied with these fears, we deal with social and relationship fears. We are afraid of being attacked emotionally, being controlled, or of being abandoned by someone we love. Even subtle put-downs or times of coldness may cause us to feel anxious. Murray Bowen (1988),[4] an important pioneer in family therapy, believes that chronic anxiety is always present in people. Anxiety affects us individually and collectively. According to Bowen, families develop rules, roles, and rituals to help each other deal with the stresses and anxieties of being in a family—and of being a family in a stressful and anxious world.

Psychological defenses, whether in individuals, families, or in larger societies, help to minimize and manage anxiety. Defenses help us cope. So having defenses isn't necessarily bad. In fact, defenses are essential for our ability to screen out most of what could possibly overwhelm us with panic or preoccupation. Imagine if you were fully conscious, at every moment, of all that could possibly happen to you and everything that could possibly go wrong. The resulting anxiety would control your every move and wear you down physically and psychologically. Defenses are essential for keeping us fairly sane and helping us to stay on task and manage life.

But defenses can cause problems. They can get in the way of relating to one another. Defensiveness contaminates communication and causes people to get angry, stop listening, interrupt, attack, become selective in what they hear, or withdraw emotionally or physically. Defenses create confusion, frustration, and worse. In the extreme, defenses cause obsessions, delusions, destructive behaviors, and other severe forms of emotional illness. Fortunately, for most people, psychological defenses are not nearly as severe, and with practice, one can learn to successfully manage them. In very simplistic terms, psychological defenses seem to come in two broad categories: *fight* and *flight* (*freeze*, in my mind, falls under the flight category). Blaming, scolding, interrupting, yelling, controlling, or trying to browbeat with "logic" are examples of *fight* defenses. Avoiding, evading, complying, withdrawing, and emotional coldness are examples of *flight* defenses. Certainly, *flight* defenses can have their own particular ways of attacking and controlling another person. When someone storms out of a room, slams the door, and shouts an obscenity, that behavior looks and feels more like fight than flight. And the manner in which one fights, if it is simply intellectually sparring, is probably just disguised flight. So it can be unclear which defense is which. The important thing to know is that defenses, whether fight or flight, exist to minimize the threat of harm or pain. Unfortunately, getting defensive can cause harm or pain to someone else. Whether one is being *overtly* controlling by scolding and criticizing or *covertly* controlling by avoiding the person or situation, the effect is still the same. People are hurt and scared when they are attacked and hurt and scared when they are abandoned.

A typical argument is characteristically carried on by defenses; the human beings behind those defenses are powerless, for a time, to manage their runaway emotions. I frequently refer to this as a "tennis match." You know you're being defensive when you are *intent* on winning your point. You aren't being curious about what the other person is trying to say, you can't wait for your turn, you are tempted to interrupt, your body feels tense, and you feel like raising your voice or

---

4   Goldenberg, I., & Goldenberg, H. (2004). *Family Therapy*, p. 186.

leaving the room. When you can successfully manage your defenses, conversations and even arguments will feel more like you're "playing catch" than playing tennis. Talks will be more *cooperative* and less *competitive*. The goal will be less about winning one's point and more about allowing both people in the room to feel heard, understood, and accepted. I'm not saying that "tennis" can't be fun. Arguments can be enjoyable forms of intellectual sparring and frequently very illuminating when done respectfully with openness and goodwill. But people need to be very careful to end the "fun" when tension mounts and feelings are being hurt. If you decide to argue, keep the argument to 20 minutes (yes, that's possible). Everything that needs to be said can be said in 20 minutes. Be respectful. Avoid bad language and disrespectful comments.

We can't do away with defenses altogether; they are too important to us. We can, however, learn to control our defenses better. We can manage to suspend them when we need to really listen to someone and hear what they are feeling and trying to say. *The whole point of effective communication is learning to manage one's defenses in order to successfully hear and be heard.* Here is a list of some typical fight defenses and some common flight defenses. Which are your favorites?

There are certainly many other forms of psychological defensiveness—of evading the difficulty of feeling feelings. Here are some examples: drug or alcohol addiction, compulsive house cleaning, romantic affairs, preoccupation with any activity such as computer games, golf, romance novels, TV sports, shopping, cars, money, exercise, or one's physical appearance can all be forms of medicating or avoiding difficult emotions and the work of creating deep and meaningful relationships. Any activity can be pushed to preoccupying extremes that distract one from what is truly important. And any behavior that is able to alter one's biochemistry can become potentially addictive.

FIGHT DEFENSES/FLIGHT DEFENSES

accusing	withdrawing
threatening	ignoring
parenting	silence
scolding/lecturing	insincere complying/agreeing
name-calling	doing "poor me"
insinuation	being passive/aggressive
labeling	passivity
problem-solving	coldness
analyzing	justifying
sarcasm	passing the buck
filibustering	forgetting
dumping	being too "reasonable"
attacking	leaving/avoiding
gender bashing	changing the subject
dredging up the past	staying busy
labeling	minimizing
criticizing	placating
raising your voice	hiding true feelings

What other psychological defenses would you add to the list above? A good exercise to do with your couple is to copy the defense list above and have them check the defenses they use most often and then discuss the exercise in therapy. The exercise will hopefully convey each person's willingness to be open about his or her defensive habits and willingness to work on them. A good measure of a growing relationship is a couple's commitment to confessing when they have been defensive, asking for forgiveness, and increasing their commitment to being real, being fair, being open, and being patient with each other as they both grow into more mature and loving human beings.

To help couples recognize their conditioned defenses as well as their different ways of relating to each other, I often use and teach Eric Berne's[5] Parent, Adult, Child model. It's a very easy model to understand and remember. Using Berne's model is an excellent way to help people get a much clearer picture of the choices they have in speaking, listening, and relating to each other in non-defensive ways. As with other models I suggest, it may seem simplistic. But simple models are easy to remember, and when someone is upset, it's good to have skills that are easy to remember and easy to use.

The Parent, Adult, Child Model

Berne's model has been around for more than 60 years—a long time by today's standards.

Berne called his model transactional analysis. By that he meant having a model with which to understand how we relate to each other and how to be more conscious of our options to speak or listen from our "parent," "adult," or "child" ego states. His most famous book, *Games People Play* (1969), became part of our pop culture. Berne popularized the concepts of being "parental," "playing games," and "getting in touch with one's inner child." Pop jargon or not, it's a very useful model. I like its simplicity, teachability, and usefulness in helping people look at the different ways they interact with each other.

Briefly, the model suggests that each person has an inner parent, the voice in one's head that reminds us of the things we *should* do; a child, which constitute our *wants* and *needs*; and an adult that arbitrates between parent and child. I've described these three ego states below.

I'm very aware of the argument between the disciplined parent in me and the less disciplined child. When I walk into a store that sells coffee, I immediately hear from my inner child who wants a muffin along with my coffee. My inner parent immediately scolds the child reminding him that coffee is enough, and we don't need a muffin. I try not to make a scene in the store while the two of them have their internal argument. Frequently the child wins.

Parent

Berne suggests that there is a parent in each of us which corresponds to our internal messages of should and must. These are the thoughts and feelings that signal an obligation, a task or responsibility, or even a prescribed way of thinking or feeling about a situation. We often find ourselves feeling guilty or ashamed when

---

5   Berne, E. (1961). *Transactional Analysis in Psychotherapy.*

we ignore the voice of our inner parent. We learned to feel that way as children, typically in order to help us regulate our safety, health, and responsibilities. Ideally, these "social emotions" provide valuable clues to appropriate behavior in certain social situations. Alternatively, people often suffer from a too severe and rigid critical parent—a merciless inner voice that relentlessly shames and criticizes. The shaming and blaming can be focused on oneself or projected outward onto others. It's also very important to have access to internal messages that correspond to one's inner nurturing parent. Having an adequate nurturing parent within, one hears messages of grace and self-acceptance. Ideally, one's internal critical parent reminds us of appropriate behaviors without creating feelings of shame and guilt. And one's nurturing parent is the reassuring, humanizing voice we hear when we make a mistake.

Child

The child inside corresponds to our wants, our needs, and frequently, our wounds. A healthy inner child is spontaneous, creative, imaginative, and playful. The healthy inner child needs fun, friends, and free time. He or she brings innocence, wonder, and enthusiasm to life and wants to experience love, acceptance, and joy. Armed with the resilience and faith of this inner child, people have the vitality and inner resources to face life's challenges. Unfortunately, too few people have an especially healthy inner child.

No one escapes childhood without being wounded in some way. Sometimes those wounds are specific or recurring traumas. Sometimes the environment in which people grow up is itself traumatic. Childhood wounds do not need be traumatic, however, to affect one as an adult. A "pleasant" home life, for example, can be stiflingly repressive. Spoken and unspoken family rules exist to keep everything "pleasant." In these homes, "nice" is the supreme ethic. The victims of such an environment are *honesty*, *authenticity*, and *vulnerability*. Growing up in the "nice factory," one learns to guard one's true feelings, one's honest perceptions, and, unfortunately, one's authentic self.

So whether emotional wounding occurs as a result of traumatic experiences in childhood or by the unhealthy family environment in which one is raised, no one escapes childhood without some emotional consequences. Childhood experiences form the basic emotional learning that influences our adult relationships. Research has convincingly shown that the nature of one's early attachments becomes the template from which one experiences and responds to all subsequent relationships. The emotional conditioning of childhood can impact one in many surprising ways. In the grip of an emotionally intense situation, people may find themselves feeling or behaving like a child. They can fly into rages, throw tantrums, pout, or act out with money, food, alcohol, or other types of immature behaviors. Worse yet, people can be raised with certain values and expectations that may condition them to think, feel, and continue to behave in very immature ways.

Adult

Being a grown-up is not synonymous with being an adult. The main difference between an adult and a child is the ability to choose wisely. Children typically cannot choose how to respond to their emotions. Adults can (or should be able to). In our Parent, Adult, Child model, the adult part of the personality is our awareness of alternative ways of thinking, feeling, and behaving, and the ability to *respond* to situations rather than to simply *react* to them. A psychologically healthy adult is conscious of the wants and needs of the inner child as well as the *shoulds* of the inner parent—and can negotiate trade-offs between those two ego states. In this way, effective adult functioning enables one to balance obligation and recreation, balance energy *in* and energy *out*, and be more capable of wise and loving choices in relationships.

Every day, I negotiate trade-offs. There are many things I enjoy that take too much time, cost too much, or are fattening. I also know that I am very fortunate to even have these choices. Many people don't. But, because I have these options, I try to make responsible decisions for myself and others—to be in the world in a thoughtful, disciplined way. Being wise, considerate, and conscious may not be the most popular virtues. But that's what it takes to have mature adult functioning.

Another characteristic of healthy adult functioning is the ability to turn the other cheek. As I explained above, when faced with a painful accusation or attack, a mature individual will step back from a defensive *reaction* of fight or flight and stay in the painful or difficult situation long enough to take a deep breath, think for a moment (or longer if necessary), ask for wisdom from within, and wisely *respond* to the attack. The choice may be to considerately *confront* or courageously *accept*. The hallmark of mature, adult functioning is the *ability to be conscious of those options and to choose wisely*. Interestingly, in order to genuinely accept something or someone, one must have the *ability* to confront. Otherwise it isn't a true choice; it's just what one does—passive acceptance. And for someone to be able to genuinely confront, one must have the *ability* to be accepting. Otherwise it isn't a true choice; it's just what one does—get upset and react angrily. There's a tremendous difference between a loving confrontation and "going off" on someone. There is a tremendous difference between wise acceptance and a cold or cowardly withdrawal. These later choices require maturity and discipline. Practicing these choices creates growth. I'll repeat again that it isn't enough to read how to communicate from a book; the lessons must be rehearsed and put into action.

In this next chapter I describe a typical case in couple therapy and illustrate the steps necessary to help them. I can't imagine a more powerful illustration of the dynamics of a narrative system than that existing in a marriage or other committed relationship. A systems perspective centers around the notion of "circular causality"—how the elements of a system interact with each other to produce or discourage change. The narrative aspects in these relationships center around the stories that each partner projects onto the relationship. In a typical relationship, his story is created from his past experience interfacing with his present experience and, modified by the same dynamics existing in his partner's story, her story is co-constructed by its interaction with her partner's story. Couples live inside of these stories, and modifying or extracting themselves from an entrenched and well-traveled storyline requires tremendous effort by both the couple and the therapist.

The first step in therapy is always to listen carefully. You'll recall the advice Carl Rogers gave: listen empathically, accept unconditionally, and be genuine. You'll then ask questions to make sure that you understand the problems the couple is facing. You'll form some tentative hypotheses about the couple's level of maturity, motivation, and insightfulness; about their communication challenges and defenses; and the specific problems the couple wants to work on. You'll then clarify and jointly agree on goals for therapy. In the back of your mind you anticipate that the main problem the couple is having is their difficulty communicating with each other and negotiating behavioral change. If they could do that, they would likely not be sitting in front of you. That's not always the case, however. Some couples can communicate fine, but they need advice on how to launch an adult child still living at home or weigh the pros and cons of placing a child in private school. There may be any number of issues that a couple might seek therapy to discuss, but it's likely that the main focus of couple therapy will be to learn and practice skills.

Questions for Discussion

1. How would you characterize your inner parent?
2. How would you characterize your inner child?
3. What are typical conflicts between your inner parent and inner child?
4. Do you recall you father ever being child-like?
5. Do you recall you mother ever being child-like?
6. What parental messages were modeled for you?
7. Did you see much evidence of "adult" functioning in your parents?

CHAPTER NINE

The Story of Relationships

CHAPTER SUMMARY AND LEARNING OBJECTIVE

Chapter 9 begins with a typical couple conflict. Jim and Julie are arguing about their son, Matt. Their argument illustrates some of the most common conflict areas in relationship, their typical fight/flight defenses, and dysfunctional conflict styles. The chapter focuses on the difference between *content* and *process* and the vital role the therapist plays in helping clarify issues, point out defenses, interpret emotions, and moderate conflicting perspectives. The therapist also identifies differences in personalities, styles of communication, conflict patterns, and the typical "circular causality" that intensifies and distorts difficult conversations.

The learning objective for this chapter is to describe typical couple conflict styles and patterns.

A Counseling Session

Jim and Julie are sitting in front of you looking anxious. This is their first appointment for marriage counseling. They've been married 19 years and have two children, a daughter 13 and a son 15. They both seem to be in good shape—Jim in slacks and a golf shirt, and Julie in a jogging outfit. In the waiting room they looked over and signed the informed consent and limits of confidentially forms. Before you have a chance to ask them what prompted their call to you, Julie exclaims, "We've been arguing a lot lately and I think we need a separation. Jim wanted to try counseling first and I agreed, but I think things have gone too far." "What do you mean by too far," you ask. "I found marijuana in our son's backpack and told his father. I didn't want to tell him because I knew what would happen. When Jim came home from work, he confronted Matt; they screamed at each other for about 15 minutes and Matt left the house. That was three days ago, and he hasn't come home yet." "What do you mean he hasn't come home?" Jim said angrily, "He came home the next day to get his stuff and you let him in!" "Of course I let him in," Julie replied, "he needs his backpack for school and some clothes." "And that's the problem, in a nutshell!"

Jim exclaimed, "My wife enables our son to walk all over us. He uses drugs, he's never home, his grades are in the toilet, and all Julie does is make excuses for him." "He hates being here," Julie said, "all you do is criticize him. No wonder he's depressed. I'm depressed too for that matter. I just need to get away from you for a while." They both became quiet. It's not hard to see the circular causality with this couple, each blaming the other in a regressive cycle that has polarized them into a painful standoff. You decide to check out this initial hypothesis. "How long have you been arguing about your son?" you ask. "Since he turned 15," Julie replied, "and started hanging out with his friends, Josh and Chris." "Did you argue much before then," you ask. "Yes, but not so much about Matt. Jim tends to be critical; he's always been hard on the kids." "Only when I need to be," Jim interjected. "And, at the same time, I attended all of Matt's little league games and Megan's soccer games. I even coached her team for a while. The kids know that I love them. I'm only hard on them when I need to be." "And I usually back him up," Julie said, "but his way of dealing with Matt isn't working anymore and he won't listen to anything I say." "What other things do you frequently argue about?" you ask. "Right now, most things," Jim said. "I don't like to argue," Julie said. "And that's why you keep giving in to Matt!" Jim exclaimed. Listening to Jim and Julie argue is painful, not just because they are hurting each other but because their lack of *process* (communication) skills makes it impossible for them to successfully discuss the *content* or issues that need to be resolved. You'll notice this dynamic from one couple to the next. By the end of your first session you will have observed the issues that have brought them into therapy as well as their lack of process skills, the differences in their temperaments, the different ways they manage stress, and the nature of the circular causality that keeps them stuck. You will also notice their levels of motivation, emotional maturity, and capacity for insight.

You ask them if their arguing has gotten worse lately and Julie responds, "The past few months have been really bad. We can't talk about anything without arguing. Jim complains about money, the house, the kids—it seems like he's never happy." "I work hard for every dollar I make," Jim interrupts, "is it too much to ask my wife to be careful about her spending or that the house be reasonably picked up when I get home?" "I *am* careful about spending!" Julie interrupts, "And no one would say that the house is messy! Why do you have to be so picky and critical?"

Unfortunately, this first session with Jim and Julie is typical of the initial sessions that you will have with many of your couples. When a couple decides to see a marriage counselor it's either because they're having serious trouble talking to each other and working things out, or something bad has happened, or both. Yes, it's great when a couple decides to get counseling before things get bad, either because they're planning a wedding or because they simply realize that marriage can be difficult and they want to have the skills to make sure it works. But this isn't the norm. When I get a call from someone wanting counseling, it's frequently urgent and usually because the couple knows that things won't get better without help. I know that it's hard for many couples to make that first appointment. For some, it feels like they've failed in some way. Others may be afraid of what the therapist might find out, or say, that could make things worse. And some couples are just nervous about change. I'm still a bit surprised, now that therapy is much more acceptable, that couples are still waiting to see a therapist until things are really bad or as a last-ditch effort to avoid divorce.

Yes, it's a good idea to see a therapist to try to avoid divorce, but why wait until then? I can't tell you how many times my wife and I (she's a therapist also) hear couples exclaim, "I wish we had seen you 10 years ago." What feels tragic to my wife and I is knowing that couples might have avoided so much pain and heartache if they had taken the time to learn some basic relationship skills years ago. It's also very sad that some couples wait until it's too late to get the help they need.

Content and Process

Most of the couples you'll see will complain that they can't talk to each other without arguing. They'll say that they're either fighting constantly and bickering or resigned to not bringing up certain topics and avoiding each other. Occasionally, one partner will complain about the other's constant nagging or parenting or avoiding and withdrawing. These couples are illustrating the most common types of defensive patterns in communication—the "fight" or "flight" defenses that were discussed previously. You'll likely notice one of the three common conflict patterns right away: fight–fight, fight–flight, or flight–flight. Fight–flight is probably the most common of these conflict patterns. One person in a relationship may be more extraverted or simply more invested in changing the other person and will tend to be more vocal. His or her partner may respond to feeling scolded or parented by avoiding the conversation and emotionally withdrawing. These two typically defensive communication patterns in a relationship will frequently create a *regressive cycle*. Worse than a vicious cycle, which is bad enough, a regressive cycle is a type of *circular causality* in which one person's defensive reaction creates additional stress for the other, and so forth. So that, adding to the initial stressor, whatever the couple is arguing about, there is the secondary stressor of increasing frustration about not being able to talk to each other with getting defensive, thus, making communication impossible.

Like many couples, Jim and Julie were prone to falling into this type of regressive cycle. While many males report that they dislike conflict and would prefer not arguing with their spouse, females will sometimes be the ones choosing to avoid conflict. Even if they disagree with their husbands they would prefer not provoking an argument and may simply become quietly compliant. This is what you've noticed in Jim and Julie's communication style. Julie would begin to talk and before long Jim would chime in to correct a part of Julie's story that, in his mind, she got wrong. Even if it wasn't to correct her, Jim would interrupt to explain why something happened the way it did in order to "clarify" his intentions. Julie would become quiet until Jim finished. She was very aware that interrupting, on her part, could lead to a heated argument. These three typical conflict patterns aren't in concrete with all couples, or with any couple all the time. Sometimes a person who is frequently inclined to "speak up" can get to a point of frustration where he or she "gives up." At other times the person who tends to avoid conflict will suddenly boil over with unexpressed frustrations. So don't make the mistake of imagining that the conflict pattern you see before you is actually typical for this couple. There are situations where the pattern may change radically. For the most part, however, understanding typical conflict patterns in relationships is very useful for suggesting guidelines to make the communication process go much more smoothly.

You might be tempted, too soon, to encourage one person to speak up and the other to clam up. Resist the temptation. Some therapists make the mistake of confronting a couple too early in therapy. Every book you've read on techniques of counseling has encouraged you to make sure your couple feels safe to express themselves in the early part of therapy.

Recall, again, Carl Rogers' three tenants of unconditional positive regard, empathic listening, and genuineness. In time, you'll have plenty of opportunities to be more directive, but your first therapeutic goal is to create safety and clarify issues. You want to provide your couple with the safety and acceptance they need to trust that you will be a safe and unbiased person to talk to—and this will help you minimize the risk of losing them too early in treatment. Naturally, if one person is dominating the conversation or if the intensity of their arguing becomes painful and unproductive, you'll want to gently, or sometimes firmly, encourage them to take turns—you'll remind them that you want to get to know how each person experiences their relationship. So as your couple talks to you and to each other, make a note of the *content* issues they want to work on as well as their *process* challenges. File away, for now, your observations of the work each person needs to do individually.

From your training in attachment theory, object relations theory, and family systems theory, it will soon be obvious in what ways your couple is reenacting dynamics from childhood and earlier relationships and how that reenactment plays out in their day-to-day and long-term conflicts.

Let's return, briefly, to the typical defensive patterns you'll see in most interpersonal relationships. We've already illustrated the common fight–flight pattern that Jim and Julie are stuck in. The other two common defensive patterns are fight–fight and flight–flight. The fight–fight pattern is clearly the most entertaining. I tend to schedule these folks for later in the afternoon or evening to help me stay awake. This couple comes in arguing and they keep it up until you signal them to take a break so you can focus on one person at a time—good luck with that. In the typical childish tug of war between angry partners, you'll very quickly hear most of their content issues as well as their process challenges within the first few minutes of the session.

The opposite of the fight–fight style is flight–flight. You'll rarely see the flight–flight communication pattern. It's not hard to guess why. This couple doesn't want to talk about anything uncomfortable. They avoid difficult topics and avoid each other in the meantime. Maybe they play golf together and go to the movies, but this is the couple you see in a restaurant eating their meal and not saying a word. They're going through the motions of being married, but they haven't done the hard work of facing uncomfortable feelings, learning to be open and vulnerable, and building safety and trust into their relationship. The result of this couple's avoidance is that they may be comfortable with each other, but their hearts aren't married. They won't be coming to counseling unless something happens to force them into it.

Sometimes the problems that force couples into therapy are urgent. They're losing their home, someone is severely depressed and hasn't been able to find work, a child is failing in school or is desperately ill. In these situations, you'll obviously focus on content—the problem or crisis the couple is facing. But this is not the usual reason couples present for therapy. Most of the time, the content *is* the process. In other words, their inability to discuss anything without turning it into an argument has become the major challenge of their relationship.

You can see this very clearly in the struggle between Jim and Julie. They are constantly arguing about how to deal with their 15-year-old son, Matt. Matt is uncooperative at home, has mediocre grades at school, and a poor attitude. Like most 15-year-olds, he wants to spend most of his time playing video games and hanging out with his friends. His parents are frustrated because nothing they do seems to make any difference in Matt's attitude and behavior. In their minds, this is clearly a content issue. When you ask them what types of discipline they've tried with Matt, and how successful they are as a couple discussing the situation, a very different picture begins to emerge.

Jim believes in a firm hand, clear consequences, and not negotiating Matt's responsibilities. These are important parenting values and, when administered consistently and lovingly, help to create character and good work habits in a young person. Julie, however, is concerned about Jim's approach to disciplining their children. She frequently notices Jim applying consequences in an angry and sometimes mean-spirited way. She is also alarmed about his frequent use of profanity, which she believes conveys a meta-message to the kids that *they*, not just their behaviors, are bad. To protect his fragile feelings of self-worth, Matt has gotten into the habit of tuning his father out, which obviously makes their relationship worse.

Julie doesn't openly engage or defy Jim's discipline, but her frequent efforts to salve her son's ego with comments like, "you know how your father is," has the effect, Jim complains, of not supporting his discipline. Moreover, Julie tends to be more lax in her discipline when Dad isn't home; therefore, Matt's perception that Dad's expectations are unreasonable is reinforced. Clearly, their inability to work together continues to further polarize them. As you listen to the *content* of this couple's conflict, you can immediately see that their inability to resolve their polarization is due to their lack of *process* skills and the maturity to be open to the corrective influence of each other's approach. It makes sense that when two parents are able to work together to discuss, negotiate, and integrate their values, their children stand the best chance of feeling loved and valued, as well as developing good discipline and qualities of character. And because they can't work successfully together to negotiate these values, their children are confused and frustrated. So while the initial conversations may focus on content issues, you know that what they need are process skills.

Pointing out this couple's process problem is not especially difficult. You turn to Jim and ask him, "Is it important to you that your kids know that you love them and that they are valuable human beings?" Jim is about to do his typical "Yes—but," when you turn to Julie and ask her, "Is it important to you that Matt and Amy learn good work habits, responsibility, and develop good qualities of character?" After Julie says, "Of course," you go on to say, "So the problem isn't with what you both want for your children, but how to work together to achieve these goals." "That's exactly the problem!" Jim interrupts, "Julie doesn't support me."

Your response to Jim's challenge is to clarify, "Like you, it seems that Julie loves her children and wants them to understand that just because they might behave badly at times, this doesn't mean that they are bad kids. In that respect, she genuinely *is* supporting you, but maybe not always in the best way. What I'd like to focus on is how successful the two of you are in talking to each other and working together to find solutions." You turn to Julie and ask, "If you were nervous about bringing something up to Jim, why would that be?" "I don't like conflict," she says, "and Jim would argue with me about whatever I wanted to tell him anyway." Turning to Jim, you ask, "Jim, if you choose not to bring up something to Julie why would that be?" "Because it wouldn't do any good; she would either argue with me or just ignore what I had to say and do whatever she wants." "So you're both avoiding some of the most important conversations of your life and your marriage.

And what's interesting to me is that if I were to ask each of you what would help you to actually talk to each other, your answers would be the same—you'd tell me that you would like to be able to finish discussing your thoughts without being interrupted and you'd like to get some kind of response from your partner that he or she was willing to listen to your feelings or ideas. You might think that arguments are caused by people not agreeing with one another, but it's possible to have a very useful conversation about topics that you don't agree on without fighting. Most arguments occur when neither person feels confident that they're getting their point across. And when your partner opposes your ideas with his or her own, you now have two speakers and no listeners and escalating frustration and tempers because no one feels heard."

In talking with Jim and Julie, it's easy for me to find myself lecturing—useful in the classroom, but I have to be careful not to overdo the "psychoeducation." So I try to interject some humor when appropriate, to lighten the mood. I'll bring up a funny exchange I once heard between former clients. I'll call them Mike and Linda, for example, obviously not stating their real names: "We argue a lot," Mike said, "and Linda disagrees with everything I say." "I do not!" Linda exclaimed. "I only disagree when you're wrong." "Which is all the time, according to you," Mike said. Linda was quiet. "See," she said, "I'm not disagreeing."

Arguing about arguing, Mike and Linda succeed in illustrating both their content and process simultaneously. For me, content is much less important than process. That's because it isn't usually *what* couples argue about that causes problems in marriage, but *how* they argue. Clearly, everything in a relationship needs to be negotiated, so it's natural that disagreements will occur. Easily or not, intentionally or reflexively, couples make deals about every facet of their relationship. Couples make deals about money, time, roles and responsibilities, in-laws, sex, kids, holidays, bed time, free time, and whether to order pizza or Chinese. Some deals are made quickly and effortlessly. They just seem to happen automatically. Other deals may be fought over for years and never be fully resolved. I don't necessarily recommend this book, but the title perfectly describes a core challenge in relationships: *Do I Have to Give Up Me to Be Loved by You?* (2002). The book highlights one of the most common struggles in marriage: how much of my spouse's values and ways of being do I accommodate without giving up what's important to me?

Because disagreements are normal and the *content* of *what* couples argue about is very similar from one relationship to another, I'm much more interested in the *how*—the *process* a couple uses to discuss feelings, make deals, and resolve issues. Process problems are usually what bring couples into therapy. When efforts to discuss feelings and resolve issues don't work, things get worse. Why worse? Because when you can't talk to each other without getting defensive, bringing up old hurts, and getting frustrated with each other, it can feel pretty hopeless. Couples will try to manage these feelings of hopelessness by not bringing things up and avoiding issues. It doesn't work. Like it or not, buried hurts and angry feelings may surface in sarcasm, rages, criticism, sometimes depression, and sometimes physical illness. Remember that "you cannot *not* communicate"; the communication will either be direct and responsible or indirect and ineffective. So couples need to learn the skills to be direct and open in their communication.

You will certainly spend time listening to the issues they want to resolve and perhaps make some suggestions when appropriate. But you'll have to be careful not to find yourself arbitrating their weekly arguments or getting too embroiled in their content issues instead of helping them to get the tools they need to talk to each other more successfully. Once they've learned and practiced those skills, they can address their content issues on their own. The old adage about teaching someone how to fish comes to mind. Once your couple has learned their communication skills, rehearsed them in your office, and can use their skills successfully at home to talk about feelings and resolve issues, your role as their therapist has been accomplished. If you've done a good job with your couple, your reward is to become redundant.

Many couples will find it strange that they need training in communication. "We talk just fine!" one husband insisted, "Our problem is that we don't agree! Aren't you supposed to tell us which one of us is right?" he asked. "While I'm not opposed to offering my opinion in certain cases," I replied, "my job isn't to mediate, but to educate. I want to help you develop the ability to talk to each other without getting defensive and argumentative, and for most human beings, that isn't easy. It requires learning and practicing skills."

I'll sometimes suggest that rather than using the term "communication training," it would be even more accurate to use the term "relaxation training." "You will be learning how to manage your emotions so that you're much less likely to become defensive and competitive. You and your spouse will work together, taking turns being the speaker and the listener.

You will talk about your own feelings and not blame or accuse the other person. You'll give each other feedback so that you both feel heard and understood. You are practicing being vulnerable, being open and accepting, and being safe. You'll learn to keep it short. You'll get into the conversation and get out again in one piece."

"What good will that do?" someone will ask, "How do you get anything resolved?" My reply is that you need to be able to do three things to have a happy marriage: share feelings, make deals, and have fun. But before you know what deal or deals to make, it's good to understand the underlying emotions involved. We'll talk more about emotions later. For now, it's important to know that emotions tell us what is and isn't working and motivate us to take action. If you're not aware of which emotions you're feeling or what they're up to, emotions have a way of getting in the way. Emotions can bully us into conflicts we don't really need to have. Sometimes emotions go into hiding and we find ourselves withdrawing from people we love. Many conflicts could easily be resolved if people managed their emotions more maturely. It isn't overly idealistic to say that most issues in marriage can be resolved just by talking *constructively* about how you both feel. In my marriage, for example, knowing how my wife feels about an issue helps me to be more aware and considerate. And if we find that we do need to make a deal about something, knowing that my wife cares about how I feel helps me to be more motivated to find a deal that we can both live with. My wife and I agree that eight out of ten couples seeking therapy tell us that they rarely talk to each other without arguing, and they need help learning to communicate without fighting. They can't resolve issues or make deals because they don't trust each other to truly care and follow through with their commitments. So again and again you'll find with most couples that the process *is* the content.

In *The Seven Principles for Making Marriage Work*,[1] John Gottman warns that communication training emphasizing active listening techniques isn't as helpful as most counselors think and that couples may experience a high relapse rate if

---

1   Gottman, J. (2000). *The Seven Principles for Making Marriage Work*.

other techniques aren't used in the therapy. I agree that communication training alone may not be helpful enough. So I use many different techniques to help couples, depending on their personalities and the problems involved. In fact, I will sometimes recommend Gottman to clients for the many useful suggestions and exercises in *Seven Principles*.

On the other hand, Andrew Christensen,[2] a professor and researcher at UCLA, considers the same research sources cited by Gottman but suggests that it may not be that communication training itself is ineffective as much as the "simplistic and naïve 'operationalizations' of communication." In other words, in Christensen's view, the *process* that therapists use to help people learn how to communicate effectively may not be as effective as it could be. This is an extremely important distinction. Here again, we'll look at process and content. *How* the therapist goes about the work of helping couples may be just as important as *what* kind of help is being offered. I'll have much more to say about this below.

Personalities

In addition to content and process, another thing you'll soon notice in your first couple session is the differences in your couple's personalities or temperaments. One person's temperament in a relationship is typically different (sometimes very different) from their partner's. Obviously, these differences create potential conflicts in each person's values, psychological defenses, and styles of communication, and need to be considered.

I've taught courses on theories of personality to MFT students at Pepperdine University for the past 16 years. One of my favorite ways to look at personality differences comes from the work of Carl Jung.[3]

He was one of the first psychologists to write extensively about how individuals differ in the ways they approach life (extroversion vs. introversion), look at things (sensing vs. intuition), make decisions (thinking vs. feeling), and prefer having things decided or left open (judging vs. perception). People have different appetites for closeness and independence, different ways of expressing and experiencing love, different values, different ways of seeing and deciding on things, and so forth. Many of the things couples argue about arise from the differences in their temperaments. It's important to understand the role that those different personalities played in your couple's initial attraction to each other, and how those differences, over time, affect their relationship for better or worse. That's another topic you'll want to look at more closely.

Problems

In this first session, in addition to listening to your couple's immediate reason for seeking therapy, you'll also want to know the various issues they typically argue about. This information will help you to get a feel for their relationship, the kinds of patterns that have developed, the typical challenges they are facing, and the best areas on which to focus attention first. I'll frequently remind couples that

2   Halweg, K., Grawe-Gerber, M., & Baucom, D. (eds.). (2010). *Enhancing Couples*, p. 34.
3   Jung, C. (1971). *Psychological Types*.

each relationship is unique, and that it's important for me to get to know them and how each person experiences the relationship. While every couple is unique, they are also similar in many ways—like noses. We all have one; they're all different and they're all alike.

It's important to help your couple understand why they may be facing the types of problems they're facing. Because conflict typically falls into fairly predictable and recognizable patterns, you can more easily describe the typical whirlpool of circular causality that results. You can remind them that in reacting to each other's reactions, they are creating a polarizing regressive cycle that will push each other away. Couples are both different and alike. You will want to honor their uniqueness as a couple and, at the same time, reassure them that therapists have been trained to grasp the types of circular causality fairly quickly and to suspend conclusions and judgments about people and relationships until they've taken the time to carefully explore each couple's individual patterns of relating. An important difference in how couples relate to each other may be their different "love languages." Gary Chapman (1992) in his book *The 5 Love Languages* discusses the most common variety of "love languages:" words of affirmation, quality time, receiving gifts, acts of service and physical touch. You may wish to have your couple describe their primary and secondary love language to help them better understand their different ways of relating. As you conclude your first couple session, it's good to summarize what you've heard, what you've seen, and what you think will help. You don't want to minimize the difficult challenges your couple faces, but you will want to attempt to give them some hope that things can improve. A good way to do this is to make it clear that while you see the content issues they want to resolve, you also see the difficulties they're having talking with each other, and that working together to improve their process will make resolving those issues more likely. You'll clarify that you are just beginning to work together, and any assessments must be tentative until more information is gathered. Your couple will wonder if you will be able to be fair and not take sides. You'll encourage them that you're not interested in finding fault or assessing blame. Your focus will be noticing their recurring patterns of interaction and the circular causality between them. You'll remind them that an important goal of therapy will be for each to recognize his or her contribution to those patterns and how they can work more successfully together to create a healthier relationship.

Questions for Discussion

1. Do you think you would enjoy working with couples?
2. What might be difficult for you in treating couples?
3. Have you had successful relationships modeled for you?
4. Have you had successful relationships?
5. What do you think are characteristics of successful relationships?

CHAPTER TEN

The Story of Healthy Marriages

In *The Psychology of Love* (1988), R. Sternberg's research suggests that there are three qualities vital to a healthy relationship: passion, intimacy, and decision or commitment. I prefer to use the terms valuing, belonging, and enjoying. In working with couples, therapists immediately notice both the content and process of couple conflict. In most cases, process problems can be pointed out and addressed and couples can learn to more successfully approach their content issues. At the same time, therapists assess the couple's ability to *value* each other. In *The Seven Principles for Making Marriage Work*, Gottman discusses the lethality of contempt in marriage as a predictor of potential divorce. Contempt is the opposite of the ability to value another as "other." Over time, an increasing sense of *belonging* can repair attachment deficits and enable individuals to experience a deeper sense of well-being. And, of course, enjoying one another, negotiating personality differences, values, and interests are all essential for lifelong happiness.

The learning objective for this chapter is to explain the essential components of a healthy marriage.

A Healthy Marriage

What does a healthy marriage look like? Perhaps you'd like to take a moment to ask yourself that question. How would you characterize it? What would be the top five qualities on your list? If you are in a relationship, what do you think would be on your partner's list? I doubt that you and your partner have identical lists, but I'm sure you share some ideas in common. That seems to be the norm. A classroom of students will arrive at about a dozen different ideas of what a good relationship looks like. But change the wording a bit and most of them will agree on a just few essential qualities.

Certainly, you will find many books and articles describing the qualities of a healthy relationship. In *The Psychology of Love*[1], R. Sternberg suggests three qualities vital to a healthy relationship: passion, intimacy, and decision or commitment. Obviously, it's passion that gets things going and, ideally, continues to be a vital dimension of an enjoyable relationship. Commitment—sticking with someone for better or worse—is what gives a relationship the time to create genuine intimacy. And intimacy, in Sternberg's view, is passion—plus. The "plus" is the deep quality of friendship, mutual sharing, and interdependency that couples work on and acquire over time. So enjoying a quality of commitment in which two people are able to share passion and intimacy is clearly a great relationship.

Valuing

I like the three characteristics Sternberg uses to identify a healthy relationship, but I'd like to amplify them a bit. For me, the three most important qualities in a relationship are valuing, belonging, and enjoying each other. Valuing, for me, involves more than a decision or a commitment to stick with someone. That's a good start. In my mind, valuing someone involves a daily discipline of considering *who* the other person is and behaving in ways that safeguard and enhance the other's well-being. Love, rightly understood, is extending oneself in ways that communicate value in the language of the *other*. Saying "I love you" can sometimes be confused with feeling good about someone. Truly and honestly saying "I value you" requires an awareness of who the other actually is. Knowing someone takes time and a willingness to experience who that person truly is. Clearly, lasting friendships arise from valuing another, along with knowing oneself also to be truly valued.

Belonging

The second vital quality in a relationship is *belonging*. This, for me, is the fruit of intimacy. The word "intimacy" can mean many things. One can speak of "intimate friends," "intimate moments," and "sharing intimacies." One would hope that each of those types of intimacy enhances valuing, builds trust, and creates a bond—all vital characteristics for genuine friendship. Add "sexual intimacy," ideally the only type of intimacy that can be shared singularly with one other human being, and you have the makings of the deep intimacy of feeling that you belong to each other. More than the warmth and trust of good friendship and the passions of sexual love, the sense of belonging inhabits one mentally, emotionally, and physically. The limbic connections, described in *A General Theory of Love*— limbic resonance, limbic regulation, and limbic revision—detail a progressive physiological, emotional, and mental interconnectedness in which two human beings enjoy the fullest range of attachment benefits:

> Because loving is reciprocal physiologic influence, it entails a deeper
> and more literal connection than most realize. Limbic regulation affords
> lovers the ability to modulate each other's emotions, neurophysiology,

---

[1]   Sternberg, R. (1988). *The Psychology of Love*, pp. 119–138.

hormonal status, immune function, sleep rhythms, and stability. ...
When somebody loses his partner and says a part of him is gone, he is
more right than he thinks. A portion of his neural activity depends on
the presence of that other living brain. Without it, the electric interplay
that makes up him has changed.[2]

I could certainly take more time and space to describe the physical and emotional benefits of two people feeling as though they belong to each other. And
there are plenty of poems and songs I could use as illustrations. It is enough to
say that the commitment couples share with each other is the foundation for the
openness and trust needed to create an exceptionally close friendship and sense
of belonging.

Enjoying

The third characteristic of a healthy relationship is enjoying—finding joy in the
other. When I interview a couple, I frequently ask questions such as "Do you like
each other?" and "Are you able to have fun together?" Unfortunately, too many
couples become burdened down with the responsibilities of living together—going
to work, paying bills, taking care of a home, kids, etc., and they've forgotten how
to play. People form relationships, for the most part, because they enjoy being
with each other. And if they aren't careful it becomes too easy to settle into boring
routines and forget to have fun. If you want to make sure that your relationship
stays healthy and energizing, it's vitally important that you take the extra time
and energy necessary to get out and play.

I remember a wife telling me during a counseling session "I know my parents
loved me, but I never felt as if they liked me. My husband really seems to like me,
and his having liked me for so many years has meant everything to me. I'm now
able to think of myself as a likeable person. So I've been able to be friendly and
more outgoing as a result, and I've even come to like myself." This is what can
happen in a good marriage; people can help to heal each other.

Practicing Playfulness

Sigmund Freud said that for a person to be psychologically healthy he or she would
need to be able to both love and work. Perhaps because I grew up in 20th century
Southern California instead of turn-of-the-century Vienna, it easy for me to add
another quality to Freud's list: play. Love and work can certainly be sources of
happiness and joy, but adding play gives a relationship something special, a unique
source of energy that emphasizes vulnerability and wonder. A quick way to take
the emotional temperature of a couple or family is to ask them what they do for
fun. It's sad that so many marriages fail because of a failure to balance the joy and
work of love. No doubt there is a correlation between the emotional health of a
relationship and the time couples devote to having fun together.

When I think about the concept of emotional health, I think about things like
commitment and loyalty, vulnerability and intimacy, caring and taking turns.

---

2   Lewis, T., Amini, F., & Lannon, R. (2001). *A General Theory of Love*, pp. 207–208.

But I also think about passion and playfulness. When couples are passionate and playful, they are able to access that creative energy that makes a relationship truly enjoyable and enduring. An emotionally healthy relationship should be joyful, not simply functional.

I remember a wife telling me about her firefighter husband, "He never takes off his uniform." By that she meant that he doesn't seem to be able to relax. "He's a captain at work," she said, "he's a captain with the kids, and he's a captain with me. I don't want to be married to a captain," she exclaimed. "I like that he is very organized, very reliable, and responsible. But I wish he could also be playful and silly sometimes."

It's interesting to me how many films I could list where one of the main challenges for a husband or wife was their inability to set aside being so responsible. According to the Parent, Adult, Child model I described earlier, some couples fall into the habit of one of them over functioning in his or her "parent ego state" and the other being too much in his or her "child." I can readily understand the nature of their attraction to each other. Each is attracted to the balancing attributes in the other. But dislodging them from their habitual roles in order to create a more balanced relationship may require using the the emergency device known as the "Jaws of Life."

It is possible to bring play back into a relationship. But couples need to get over being competitive with each other and practice being more vulnerable. And they can't be afraid to look or act silly. They were playful and silly at times when they first met. Hopefully they haven't become too tired, lazy, easily embarrassed, resentful, and afraid of their partner's disapproval to find time for play. But it's sad that that is often the case. Below are some simple suggestions I routinely recommend to couples for making love fun. Some of them seem very silly, but playfulness keeps the relationship fresh and enjoyable. Clearly, as a therapist, you can't make these suggestions right away. Most couples have too much work to do in therapy to get past being frustrated and competitive with each other and restore trust. Once you notice your couple responding to therapy, being less argumentative, and more willing to be vulnerable and take risks, you can make some suggestions to bring some fun back into the relationship.

Encourage your couple to begin with easy stuff that is both inexpensive and low-cal: tickle each other, go for walks, hike in the woods or hills, learn some new jokes, wrestle (good-naturedly), dance, learn to dance, go horseback riding, chase each other outside with squirt guns, give each other small fun presents, make up a treasure hunt, go to the park and swing on the swings, sing songs together, be silly sometimes, play board games, go bike riding, lay on your back and see shapes in the clouds, read to each other. For couples I suggest taking a shower together, giving each other foot rubs, neck rubs, back rubs, writing out things you like about each other, giving cards for no reason, washing each other's hair, watching *I Love Lucy* reruns, feeding each other ice cream, making a list of others things that you would enjoy and doing one each week. Take turns planning and initiating dates and outings. Take time to find out what your partner would really love to do. John Gottman has some great ideas in his book *Seven Secrets of a Happy Marriage*. I could go on and on, but you get the point.

Notice that most of the activities above seem very childish. Right! So do the mushy words that lovers call one another. When you let yourself feel too old to be silly, your relationship will become old too. Keep it fresh—make time for fun. It's okay to be "kids" with each other. Being child-like helps you to be unguarded and more vulnerable with each other and, in turn, more relaxed and loving. You are lovers, business partners in life, perhaps co-parents, and, hopefully, best friends. But don't forget that you are also playmates.

I once gave a couple a unique homework assignment. I recall that our session ended on a warm and beautiful summer evening. Their assignment was to go to the local Baskin-Robbins for an ice cream cone. I instructed them to sit on the bench just outside the store and enjoy the pleasant summer evening and eat their ice cream together. Not an especially innovative assignment, but this couple had forgotten that they once liked each other. They had forgotten that they were not just fellow laborers in the tasks of life but also playmates. They needed to be reminded to have fun.

Deals, Feelings, and Fun

Another thing that you'll want to remind your couple is that they have more than one relationship in their relationship. According to the Parent, Adult, Child model, there are six "people" in the marriage. If you consider that the "inner parent" can be both critical as well as nurturing, and that the child inside can be both playful and healthy as well as wounded and withdrawn, that means that each one of us can be in at least five different "ego states." Recall that an ego state is what we are thinking and feeling at any given moment. But I don't want to get too complicated or confusing. Let's go back to the simple idea that there are six "people" in a relationship—two parents, two adults, and two kids. That means that you have five different relationships. Why five? Because you can relate to each other parent to parent, adult to adult, child to child, and from time to time, when someone needs nurturing, you can also relate to each other from parent to child. Doing something nice for the other; taking care of your partner when he or she is sick, frightened, or discouraged; nurturing them in some important way will help your partner to feel cared for as well as cared about. There is nothing wrong with allowing oneself to feel needy and needing care at times, as long as it is reciprocal, balanced, and temporary. What doesn't work in a relationship is when one partner spends too much time in his or her "child" forcing the other to take up the slack and spend more time than is fair having to be the "parent."

Making Deals

In a healthy relationship, couples are able to make deals. Couples make deals about everything, from what side of the bed to sleep on and who unloads the dishwasher to when and how to retire and where to bury each other. Some deals are quickly and easily made, and others may take a lifetime to negotiate. My wife and I have been talking about writing a book together about our experience building two houses. We made lots of deals. We may call the book *His Way—Her Way* in order to illustrate how we arrived at many of the decisions we made, not only in building our houses, but also in working together as business partners and co-parents.

When it came to designing houses, there were things my wife cared a great deal about and I didn't. There were things I cared about, and she didn't. These were easy decisions. Fortunately, we share similar ideas about floor plans, decor, etc., so most of those decisions weren't difficult either. The tough decisions happened when we didn't agree on something that we both cared about. This, it turned out, was quite a blessing. Naturally we both felt frustrated with the other at times, but we agreed to suspend our need to get our own way and decided to pray about the decision and be patient until we could get some direction.

I won't elaborate on this point here, but too many couples are afraid to be patient and open with each other. I would much prefer reaching a decision together than getting "my way" at my partner's expense. As a result of this commitment to reaching decisions together, both of us were astonished when, time after time, a solution appeared or occurred to us that neither of us had considered before. We felt that God had a hand, not only in helping us to build our home, but also in building trust and closeness in our marriage. You don't need to be religious to build a house, but it helps to have faith—faith that the two of you are mature and adult enough to navigate through the minefield of myriad decisions, from floor plans to doorknobs, with your marriage intact.

So, to review, I've talked about the three qualities of a healthy relationship—valuing, belonging, and enjoying. I've also talked about the five relationships that exist in a relationship, parent–parent, adult–adult, child–child, parent–child in one direction, and parent–child in the other. The two "parents" in the relationship work together to make *deals*—to manage and negotiate money, time, roles and responsibilities, kids, social events, and so forth. The "kids" in the relationship find time for *play dates* and having fun. The "adults" in the relationship are friends who *share feelings* and needs and keep things balanced in the "inner family" of parents and kids. And in healthy relationships, people take time to do loving and caring things to nurture each other.

Questions for Discussion

1. What, for you, are important qualities in a relationship?
2. What do you bring to relationships that are valued by others?
3. What would be a romantic date for you?
4. What "fun" qualities would you want in your relationships?
5. What do you think is your "love language"?
6. If you are currently in a relationship, what is your partner's "love language"?

CHAPTER ELEVEN

The Story of Conflict

CHAPTER SUMMARY AND LEARNING OBJECTIVE

It's important for couples to realize that conflict is inevitable in growing relationships. Conflict occurs when values and personality differences surface and need to be resolved or negotiated. Avoiding conflict may lead to buried resentments, acting-out behavior, boredom, or stagnation. In *Looking for Spinoza*, Antonio Damasio illustrates the relationship between thoughts and feelings and the challenges humans face with difficult emotions. Those difficult emotions are activated, covertly, according to Damasio, in contexts that trigger associations with past experiences. That can be good, albeit difficult, news. As dissociated experience surfaces, often in conflict, those dissociated emotions can be integrated into conscious and adaptive functioning. For the authors of *A General Theory of Love*, "Long-standing togetherness writes permanent changes into a brain's open book. In a relationship, one mind revises another," is the hopeful outcome of couple conflict that is dealt with successfully a loving relationship.

The learning objective for this chapter is to explain the role of conflict in relationships, to normalize conflict, and to explain the healthy management of conflict for healing and growth.

Certainly, there are many different causes of conflict in relationships. Those causes can be generalized as differences in cultural and family conditioning, divergent expectations for relationships, competition for physical and emotional needs, differences in temperament, and immature and irresponsible behaviors. The purpose of this chapter is to illuminate the fundamental reasons for conflict and preview ways to manage it.

The Purpose of Conflict

Conflict exists because people compete to survive. People compete for love and attachment.

People compete for happiness and security. Sometimes conflict exists because, for various reasons, people want it to. I will likely say this more than once: *trying to eliminate all conflict in a relationship is a bad idea*. Growing from conflict is a much better goal. Conflict is inevitable and even desirable for reasons we will discuss below. The idea is to understand the role conflict plays in relationships and the means to grow from it. That's one of the most important goals of therapy.

In order to fully understand and grow from conflict one needs to appreciate the biological basis for conflict. That involves understanding the role that emotions play in creating psychological defenses, and the extremely significant role of early childhood conditioning and attachments. I plan to go into this in much more detail below, but first let's look at the important role that conflict can play in relationships.

People frequently imagine that having conflict means that the relationship is in trouble. On the contrary, a *conflict-free* relationship is usually an indication of trouble. Having no *visible* conflict in a relationship is often a sign of boredom, apathy, lack of trust, or resignation. If conflicts are not visible, they are usually invisible—felt but not managed, and certainly not resolved. Good relationships typically benefit from conflict handled responsibly and fairly.

Conflict is an inevitable part of the process of growing and of a growing relationship. And because people are different, and those differences make up a large part of attraction, occasional conflict is often part of the deal. Consequently, it's very important not to try to eliminate all conflict but to develop the skills necessary to understand, manage, and learn from conflict.

Among the tasks of energizing close interpersonal relationships is negotiating the things we need and the things that make us happy. One might guess that this is where conflict begins—and it often is. However, conflict exists *inside* of people as often as *between* people. A decision to sit down and read, for example, is a trade-off between reading and the many other more enjoyable or less enjoyable tasks that one might choose. A typical day for fortunate people consists of many such conscious and unconscious trade-offs—negotiations between the things that we need to do or should do and other things that we might prefer. Some of these trade-offs are quite easy while others require a great deal of self-awareness and discipline.

We often become confused about what our deepest needs are; they evolve as we grow and mature. A good relationship helps us to know ourselves better, to experience our inner conflicts and demons, and, eventually, to discover what truly makes us happy. But learning and growing from conflict isn't automatic, and poorly managed conflict can be devastating. Consequently, it's essential to remember that conflict has value, conflict has a function, and conflict can be understood and managed to bring about growth.

In teaching courses on personality theories—the "what and why" of human nature—I've discovered that virtually all personality theorists agree that *outer* conflicts most commonly begin as *inner* conflicts. Inner conflicts involve, among other things, the need to feel sane, secure, and significant, and the best ways to meet those needs. Meeting those needs, however, involves other people and their needs. Conflict is the result. And this is precisely why conflict in relationships can be so important and useful—it has the potential to help us grow in our ability to be both conscious and conscientious.

So conflict can be both useful and potentially dangerous. Consequently, it's important to know how to contain and manage conflict in order to benefit from it. There are two parts to managing conflict: understanding why it exists and learning the skills to deal with it. Understanding the reasons why conflict occurs helps us to make sense of it, be less afraid of it, be less defensive, and to potentially be more accepting and even more open and curious. *Acceptance* and *curiosity* are two of the most valuable qualities to have in dealing with conflict, but just as important is learning the skills necessary to resolve conflict and grow from it.

Learning those skills is the hardest work couples can do. It's hard because it requires managing emotions—and managing emotions is much more difficult than understanding them. It's also hard because genuine learning, especially emotional management, requires a great deal of practice. There are few things about relationships that I can state as absolute fact. This is one of them. If people are unwilling to learn how to communicate wisely and lovingly, they will not have the quality of relationship that is possible for them. Regardless of how much people love each other, how well they get along, and how few conflicts they have, there are depths of love, qualities of rapport, and levels of growth that cannot be attained without developing skills.

I am almost embarrassed to harp on the importance of developing communication skills. By now, it is such a well-known, well-worn, and overused cliché that I can hardly bring myself to state so obvious a truth. But it is the truth—and a very important truth. Relationships are about relating. How people relate to each other; the quality of their openness, trust, curiosity, and acceptance; and their willingness to negotiate perceptions, values, and needs will determine the quality of their relationship. Love is a beautiful but meaningless concept without the skills of relating well. But before we go into detail about the skills necessary to manage conflict and communicate effectively, it is vital to understand that our childhood conditioning and emotional imprinting combine with our temperament to determine how we develop, who we become, who we fall in love with, and why we have the particular types of conflicts we have.

I invite you to take a close look at the visual below from Anthony Damasio's *Looking for Spinoza* (2003). I've looked at many diagrams in many texts on psychology over many years, and I don't know of one that is more useful that Damasio's construct below of the relationship between thoughts and feelings, and their impact on decision-making. A quick explanation of the illustration is to notice the tendency of the brain to quickly (and, Damasio says, covertly) create associations between present and past experience. So an event today, if it resembles an emotional experience from the past, may be intensified or distorted because of its past emotional association.

In this diagram, we see that any given event is processed both cognitively and emotionally.

Path A (cognitive processing) and path B (emotional processing) operate both independently and cooperatively. That's good news—when it isn't bad news. Everything that we've been looking at, in terms of attachment, conditioning, and other life experiences, is inside the box labeled "Covert activation of biases related to emotional conditions of comparable situations." Notice especially path B, emotional processing, and the unavoidable impact of covert activation of learned emotional bias on present decisions.

In other words, whether we like it or not and whether we are aware of it or not, our brain tends to organize experience by connecting present emotions with past events of a similar emotional quality. The more intense the present emotional event, the more likely it will activate similar past emotional experience. The good news is that our pleasant experiences can be intensified by similar experiences

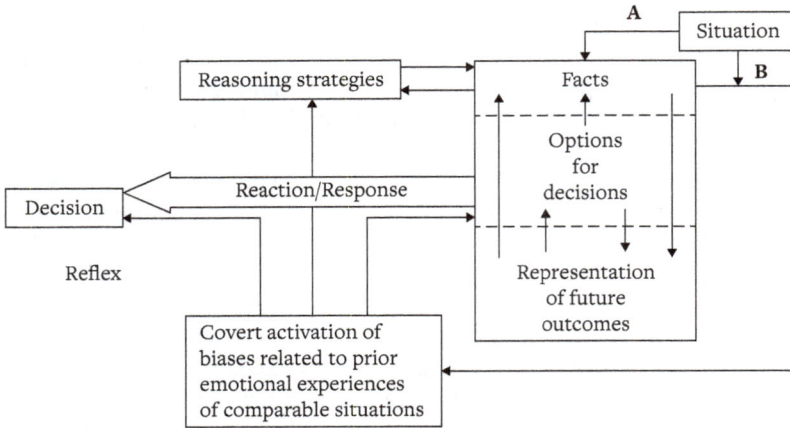

FIG. 11-1 Normal decision-making uses two complementary paths. Confronted with a situation that requires a response, path A prompts images related to the situation, the options for action, and the anticipation of future outcomes. Reasoning strategies can operate on that knowledge to produce a decision. Path B operates in parallel and prompts activation of prior emotional experiences in comparable situations. In turn, the recall of the emotionally related material, be it covert or overt, influences the decision-making process by forcing attention on the representation of future outcomes or interfering with reasoning strategies. On occasion, path B can lead to a decision directly, as when a gut feeling impels an immediate response. The degree to which each path is used alone or in combination depends on a person's individual development, the nature of the situation, and the circumstances. The intriguing decision patterns described by Daniel Kahnemann and Amos Tversky in the 1970s are probably due to engagement of path B.

Source: Antonio R. Damasio, "Thoughts and Feelings," Looking for Spinoza. Copyright © 2003 by Harcourt Inc

from the past. The bad news—I'm sure you've caught on. Which is why it isn't so easy to *just get over it!* Cognitive therapy, as I've stated above (think this way, don't think that way), can be very effective. It's the key focus of the majority of self-help books. And practicing positive thinking is an essential life skill. But the emotional content inside that box on path B is stubborn stuff. Psychotherapy can provide the means for in-depth emotional healing and transformation, but so can a *good* marriage. A good marriage will create the trust and vulnerability needed to get inside that box and create the foundation for a "corrective emotional experience"—the different emotional outcome required to heal the wounds from the past and create a quality of connection essential for great love and a deep friendship.

The human brain, as discussed above, is accustomed to experiencing and re-experiencing what it has already learned. A corrective emotional experience occurs when the brain is exposed to similar emotional contexts but with a different outcome. Over time, new neural pathways are created, and the brain is no longer immediately subject to past learning. Old stories are transformed with new narratives and happier outcomes. This is what the authors of *A General Theory of Love*[1] have termed "limbic revision":

---

1   Lewis, T., Amini, F., & Lannon, R. (2000). *A General Theory of Love*, p. 144.

Ongoing exposure to one person's (neural) attractors does not merely activate neural patterns in another—it also strengthens them. Long-standing togetherness writes permanent changes into a brain's open book. In a relationship, one mind revises another; one heart changes its partner. This astounding legacy of our combined status as mammals and neural beings is limbic revision: the power to remodel the emotional parts of the people we love, as our attractors activate certain limbic pathways, and the brain's inexorable memory mechanism reinforces them. Who we are and who we become depends, in part, on whom we love.

The narrative system of a healthy relationship not only describes but inscribes the transformative elements that maintain and enhance positive outcomes for each partner's story.

Questions for Discussion

1. In what contexts might you be vulnerable to emotions from past experience?
2. How would you describe the purpose of conflict in your own words?
3. At what point in a relationship are you most likely to experience conflict?
4. What do you typically feel and do when you are in conflict with another?
5. What have you learned from conflicts you have had in the past?

CHAPTER TWELVE

The Story About Helping Couples

CHAPTER SUMMARY AND LEARNING OBJECTIVE

Chapter 12 outlines the many treatment options available to the therapist working with couples. Because thoughts, feelings, and behaviors are all interrelated, therapy can be cognitively, behaviorally, or emotionally focused. Therapists must be well-versed and skillful in the application of each of those approaches. An *integrated* approach is an informed and artful appreciation of the best interventions to make with each individual couple. In a section of the book *Enhancing Couples*, Andrew Christensen observes that there are commonalities in each of the principal therapeutic approaches for helping couples. More effective than attempting a single approach, Christensen recommends a *unified protocol*, employing the key elements in each treatment. Therapists can develop a treatment plan that is tailor made to each couple, addressing insight, emotional management, and healthy choices and behaviors.

The learning objective for this chapter is to know the principal approaches to doing couple therapy and to explain the concept and uses of a unified protocol in treating relationships.

Your Treatment Plan

By the end of your first session you've noticed quite a lot about your couple, including the three things you need to anticipate a positive outcome. Recall that these three things are an adequate amount of insightfulness, maturity, and motivation. An adequate amount of insight or intelligence is important for people to be able to understand what doesn't work and learn to do things differently. An adequate amount of maturity is required for people to be able to manage troubling emotions and make reasonable decisions. And, obviously, without an adequate amount of motivation, we're not going anywhere. If one of these qualities is missing, therapy may not work.

Also, by the end of the first session, you've begun to mentally construct a treatment plan. A treatment plan is a way of organizing impressions and observations about your couple's relationship and thoughts about the best approach to help them reach their goals. Notice I said *their goals*. Therapy is a collaborative process. You will, no doubt, make some suggestions and point out things in their communication that aren't working. You will be giving them some exercises and homework to do. You may even suggest some reasonable goals given the nature of your couple's relationship, but, ultimately, they decide what they want to get out of therapy. This may seem a bit obvious, but your couple's investment and participation in their own therapy is essential for its success. An important phrase in the recovery movement that effectively echoes my emphasis on the importance of motivation and participation is "it will work if you work it."

Speaking of participating in directing the course of therapy, years ago, a pastor referred an older man from his congregation for therapy. I knew that the pastor was from a very conservative Christian church, so I was pleased that he felt he could trust me with one of his flock. My new client seemed a bit reserved and suspicious when he first sat down. I'm used to clients being nervous at first, and I was about ready to say something to help him relax when he firmly stated, "First off, I want to make it clear that I don't want any of that Freudian double-talk!" I was a bit surprised, but smiled and replied, "All right, then, no Freudian double-talk." I'm not even sure how to do Freudian double-talk anyway. But I thought, "Good, here's a fellow who knows what he wants (or doesn't want) from therapy."

Approaches to Therapy

Marriage counselors try to keep up with the most recent literature about relationships and relationship therapy. They will read some of the more popular self-help books in order to make intelligent recommendations to their clients. They will also try to stay current with journal articles, online resources, and books designed to help them professionally. One of the most important books for therapists on marriage therapy was published in 2010. It's an excellent collection of papers by professors and researchers in the field of marriage therapy called *Enhancing Couples*.[1]

One of these papers points out five major approaches to doing couple therapy that have been thoroughly researched and empirically tested to be effective. An important consideration in psychotherapy is that an effective treatment plan for individuals, couples, and families should be evidenced-based. This is a plan constructed from clearly defined and measurable goals, and predictable, sustainable results. Each of the evidence-based treatment approaches researched in *Enhancing Couples* differs in its focus on providing insight, changing behaviors, or transforming emotions. It makes sense that each of these treatment approaches can be effective because thoughts, feelings, and behaviors are all connected and interrelated. Addressing any one of these three human functions will affect the other two. Typically, a therapist will select a therapeutic approach based on the direction most likely to be effective. He or she will consider the types of relationship problems reported and the strengths and work areas of each of the partners and make some tentative plans on how to proceed.

---

1   Halweg, K., Grawe-Gerber, M., & Baucom, D. (eds.). (2010). *Enhancing Couples*.

Thoughts, Feelings, Behaviors

Therapists hear about many different types of problems. Some people know that they need help with their thoughts, some with their behaviors, and others with their emotions. "Why do I keep having these kinds of thoughts?" for example, or "I feel depressed and discouraged most of the time," or "I'm not able to stop what I'm doing!" These are the kinds of statements therapists hear day after day. And because thoughts, feelings, and behaviors are all interrelated, therapists are able to focus attention on the most troublesome or problematic areas and see positive results in other dimensions of the individual or relationship.

For example, in his book *Feeling Good*,[2] David Burns addresses faulty thought patterns called "cognitive distortions." Examples of cognitive distortions include "Why do I think that everyone is out to take advantage of me?" "Why do I always think that something awful will happen?" "Why can't I believe that someone could actually love me?" Burns also includes some excellent exercises to deal with these cognitive distortions in his *Feeling Good Handbook*.[3] I recommend both books to clients who are struggling with all-or-nothing thinking, globalization, negativity, personalization, catastrophizing, and other types of thought disorders. Burns correctly asserts that many types of mental distress, especially depression, are caused by faulty thoughts and beliefs. Challenging and changing these cognitive distortions and patterns of thinking will make a big difference in how someone feels and behaves.

Insight-Oriented Therapies

Two types of couple therapy—Insight-Oriented Therapy and Cognitive-Behavioral Couple Therapy—are evidenced-based approaches reviewed in *Enhancing Couples* that target faulty thinking patterns and unconscious agendas that negatively impact relationships. They focus on insight and understanding—cognitive dynamics such as assumptions of how relationships ought to be conducted, standards by which relationships are judged successful or not, expectations about roles and behaviors, and attributions of fault for failures in the relationship. The goal of these types of therapies is to correct faulty perceptions and expectations and to encourage corrective insight and understanding about how relationships can be improved. *Getting the Love You Want* by Harville Hendrix (1988) is a good example of a popular self-help book that also focuses attention on insights into the reasons why someone is attracted to their partner and why, because of the very nature of that attraction, couples have the problems they have.[4] Hendrix divides marriages into two categories, conscious and unconscious. Unconscious marriages continue to act out the tug of war of competing needs without understanding why or how to work together to meet those needs. In a conscious marriage, partners grasp

---

2   Burns, D. (1980). *Feeling Good*.
3   Burns, D. (1999). *The Feeling Good Handbook*.
4   Other books that can be used to help couples gain insight into their relationship include *Boundaries in Marriage* (Townsend & Cloud, 1999) a good source for insight into the importance of safeguarding one's own individuality and developing healthy strategies for enhancing mutuality and *You Just Don't Understand* (Tannen, 1990) written by a professor of linguistics, stressing the urgent need for insight and acceptance of the ways that males and females have been socialized to communicate differently.

the underlying logic of their attraction to each other and the healing potential of working together.[5] And while Hendrix does suggest exercises that encourage couples to change certain behaviors, his insight-oriented approach is very effective in helping partners to understand the dynamics of their relationship. He helps couples to grasp where wounds occurred growing up or in past relationships, where growth and healing can take place, and how, through deepening the quality of their friendship and acceptance of each other, they can experience increased trust, closeness, and success in their marriage. A popular approach to treatment called imago therapy, developed by Hendrix, helps couples understand how their early childhood relationships affect their present relationships.

Behavior-Oriented Therapies

Two more therapeutic approaches—Traditional Behavioral Couple Therapy and Integrative Behavioral Couple Therapy—are also reviewed in *Enhancing Couples*. These approaches focus on changing behaviors and learning the skills of mutual caring. These skills include communication training, conflict management, and focusing on specific behavioral changes such as negotiating roles and responsibilities, setting aside time for business meetings, parenting plans, "caring days," and so forth. Clearly the goal of these approaches is to create direct and immediate change in the way partners treat each other, with the additional benefit that these interventions will also improve the morale and motivation of each.[6]

There's no question that people seeking marriage therapy want to see positive changes as quickly as possible. Sometimes, the best thing a therapist can do is to assess the most immediate problems and try to determine the quickest way to create change. Asking questions such as "Why did you decide to call me?" or "What feels like the most important thing for us to work on?" may be ways of bringing these issues out into the open where they can be discussed and negotiated. It's important to deal with crisis situations immediately to relieve stress, create safety, and strengthen the motivation necessary to pursue long-term goals.

Emotionally Focused Therapy

The fifth therapeutic approach included in *Enhancing Couples* is emotionally focused couple therapy. Susan Johnson originated this well-researched approach to working with couples by stressing the importance of accessing and working through entrenched and problematic emotions. As I mentioned above, thoughts, feelings, and behaviors are all interrelated. A therapist can focus attention on any one of these areas and expect to see positive changes in the other two. Johnson affirms that in many cases altering one's cognitive distortions and modifying behaviors may be next to impossible (as noted previously) when thoughts and behaviors are

---

5   I'm not aware of any text that does a better job of explaining the neurophysiologic dynamics of attraction and healing better than *A General Theory of Love* (Lewis, Amini, & Lannon, 2000). This is a must-read for anyone doing relationship therapy.

6   Gottman, J. (1999). *The Seven Principles for Making Marriage Work;* Markman, H., Stanley, S., & Blumberg, S. (2001). *Fighting for Your Marriage*; and McKay, M., Fanning, P., and Paleg, K. (2006). *Couple Skills* are three popular books that stress the importance of concrete strategies for behaving in loving ways toward one's partner.

held hostage to intransigent emotions arising from old wounds and conditioned emotional learning.

There may have been a time in an individual's early life, for example, when expecting the worst from people was a very correct and protective expectation; being vulnerable was physically dangerous, and staying protectively angry meant survival. These entrenched, conditioned emotions are not easily erased by thinking or behaving differently. Deep-seated, often protective, emotions and defenses have to surface into awareness, be understood, healed, and transformed in order to make any real progress in becoming a healthier person and relating more lovingly toward another.

In his book *Looking for Spinoza*, Antonio Damasio[7] makes the point that the body itself may be conditioned, over time and in certain environments, to hold on to a variety of emotional states. These are the "background emotions" (as discussed previously) that Damasio is referring to. The idea that our physical, mental, and emotional lives are inseparably connected and mutually interact with each other is also echoed in *The Body Remembers* by Babette Rothschild,[8] as well as *The Body Never Lies* (2006) by Alice Miller. The point is that while insight and behavioral changes are certainly important, some individuals may require more in-depth healing of conditioned physical/emotional trauma. I have often used Damasio's visual (discussed previously) to help students appreciate that what is very difficult but essential for healing is to help patients get inside of the box that represents "the covert activation of biases related to emotional experiences of comparable situations."

Where Do We Start?—Where Are We Headed?

Marriage partners want to see changes. They want a better understanding of what's happening in their relationship. They want to feel more hopeful, cared about, and valued. Where do you start? This is only the second appointment, and there probably hasn't been much change since the last session. You may ask questions such as, "How are things? What was your week like? What stayed with you from our last session?" or "What have you been talking about since we met last?" These types of questions are ways of checking in on how your couple has been doing since their last appointment and trying to decide where to begin and what to focus on first.

It's easy to sense tension when a couple walks into your office. Did they just have a bad argument? Are they facing some kind of crisis? If so, there isn't much point doing any in-depth exploration of individual backgrounds or relationship history. That will have to come later. They won't be able to concentrate on much more than what needs to be discussed or resolved in the immediate situation. So another reason you ask "How are things?" will be to give them a chance to begin the session with whatever topic feels most urgent.

On the other hand, they might have had a pretty good week. Sometimes simply beginning the process of therapy improves things at home. It's as if they're finally

7 Damasio, A. (2003). *Looking for Spinoza: Joy, Sorrow, and the Feeling Brain.*
8 Rothschild, B. (2000). *The Body Remembers.*

doing something positive; they are taking steps to work on their relationship, and they both feel encouraged. A couple told me recently that they had a good week. I asked them "Why?" I often ask that question in order to help couples become more aware of what they may be doing that's working. They looked at each other for a minute. "Mike is trying harder to be nice!" Jan exclaimed. "No, I'm not!" Mike complained, "I always try to be nice! You're the one who's actually changed. You've been way less critical!" he said. "I'm not that critical!" Jan stated emphatically, and they continued fighting about who was the one responsible for things improving. That's an interesting twist to a typical argument, but you'd be surprised at how often couples argue that it's the other one who's working harder. That may seem counter-intuitive, but it's another manifestation of the ongoing competition in couples. Neither one wants to admit that he or she had been doing anything that needed to be changed. In reality, it's likely that both people are making small changes. It often doesn't take much—a small kindness, a compliment, letting something go, or just being a little nicer, to improve the emotional climate at home. Couples can reverse the regressive cycles of reacting to each other's reaction by making small efforts to be a little kinder or more patient with each other daily. Over time, the competitive regressive cycle may be transformed into a progressive cycle as things gradually improve.

In your second session, you'll spend a few minutes reviewing the previous week and deciding which area of the relationship to work on. You'll begin thinking seriously about a treatment plan based on your assessment of the problems you're seeing, the differences in their temperaments, their levels of maturity and defensiveness, the amount of motivation, their willingness to change, and so forth. It's very likely that if they're not in any immediate crisis, you'll want to continue to explore their issues, including their individual backgrounds. Your agenda, at this point, is to gather information to determine the best way to help your couple reach their goals, but that agenda may have to be put on hold if more immediate issues need attention.

It's challenging to navigate the best course to steer in helping couples to reach their goals. I'll use the metaphor of the compass rose again. This time, instead of illustrating the five major theoretical orientations used in therapy as I did above, I'll use the compass metaphor to illustrate specific therapeutic approaches you will be using in your sessions. For example, you can be non-directive. This is the classic style of Socratic listening which does not give direction to clients but uses the process of empathic listening to enable clients "to feel felt." Carl Rogers' (1961) research into this non-directive or "person-centered" approach confirmed that, used effectively, clients are empowered to see more deeply into their situations and find their own solutions. In one sense, all therapy (unless court-ordered) is person-centered, because the task of a therapist is to help clients reach their goals. Clearly, the opposite of non-directive therapy is to be "directive." In this type of therapy, you will take a very active role in suggesting goals and the strategies required to make changes. Cognitive and behavioral therapy tends to be very directive. As you work together with your couple you will encourage their trust and their ability to be increasingly real with each other. In a directive approach, you may challenge behaviors, confront cognitive distortions, and suggest homework for your couple to work on between sessions. The challenge in selecting a directive or non-directive approach is the ability to discern which is likely to work best with which types of clients and for which types of problems. Below are some of the approaches to consider. Once again, the mariner's compass helps you to visualize the best approach to choose.

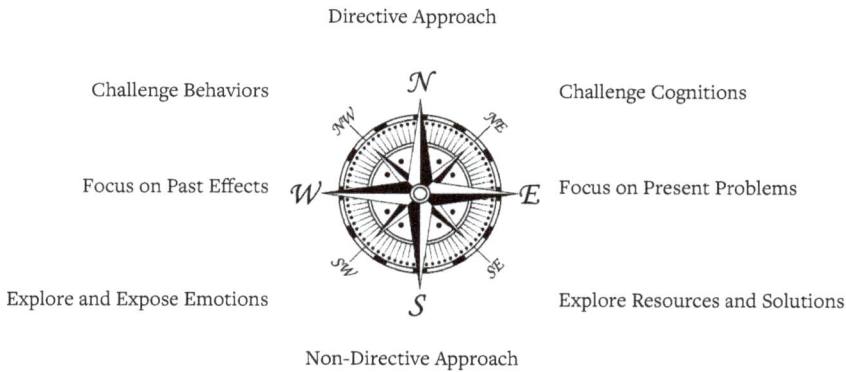

Directive Approach

Challenge Behaviors

Challenge Cognitions

Focus on Past Effects

Focus on Present Problems

Explore and Expose Emotions

Explore Resources and Solutions

Non-Directive Approach

FIG. 12-1

If your couple is facing a crisis, for example, whether the crisis is from the outside or within their relationship, you will likely be very directive and choose a behavioral approach to help them deal with the crisis in the most efficient and successful way. Once the immediate stressors are dealt with, your therapy will refocus on the insights and skills necessary for strengthening the relationship for the long haul. Other points on the compass rose may include exploring family backgrounds, reviewing childhood conditioning, any traumatic experiences growing up, and the nature of past relationships. Exploring these topics is very useful in understanding the couple's expectations of each other and why certain troubling emotions may be coming to the surface. It also makes sense to explore their relationship strengths, their social support system, and what they've survived and accomplished together. Hopefully it won't be a surprise to your couple that you will ask a lot of questions. Clearly, some "history taking" may have to be deferred to a later time in order to deal with more pressing problems in the relationship at present, but in order for therapy to be effective and lasting, you will take the first few sessions to get to know your couple and, at the same time, begin to formulate both short- and long-range treatment goals. The short-range goals will focus on resolving immediate problems, establishing safety, and building trust. The long-range goals will focus on learning the skills necessary for the ongoing challenges of living life and, ultimately, becoming better friends.

Principles of Change

Marriage and family therapists, experienced at working with couples, are bound to notice consistent recurring problems and patterns of behavior. They also learn strategies and interventions that typically work with couples. Andrew Christensen makes a good argument for moving away from focusing on one particular approach with couples and recommends that therapists employ a "unified protocol" of five effective strategies or "principles of change" common to all types of couple therapy. The advantage of focusing on these principles of change, according to Christensen, is that "it allows the clinician to concentrate on fundamental principles and their application rather than becoming certified in a plethora of treatment packages—that good clinical work requires the sensitive application of *principles* rather than dispensing techniques from various treatment *packages*."[9]

Christensen's suggestions fit very well with my own personal clinical experience. And from my conversations with other therapists, the trend today is to move away from relying solely on a single theoretical orientation in favor of skillfully integrating the principles of change common to each. It makes a great deal of sense to understand and apply the basic strategies that have been proven to be effective with couples. You will also want to make every effort to learn how and when to use which strategies with which types of relationship problems.

I'll list these five principles of change below. This will help you to organize your goals for treatment and develop an effective treatment plan. Your treatment plan will be based, in part, on the relationship strengths and weaknesses you see in your couple and the problems they want to fix. The questions you ask and the exercises you assign are based on how and when to use each of these basic strategies. You are working cooperatively with your couple to find what helps. As I've mentioned, there are many different approaches to doing couple therapy, and different approaches work better for different couples at different times. But all of these approaches share the common principles of change listed below. Christensen uses technical language to describe these strategies.[10] I'll paraphrase them for you:

Paraphrasing Andrew Christensen's Five Principles of Change

1. Develop a clear understanding of each partner's contribution to problems in the relationship, exposing the "circular causality" that reinforces ongoing conflicts.
2. Create guidelines and agreements for containing hurtful and defensive behaviors.
3. Access and clarify emotionally charged issues and behaviors; encourage vulnerability, empathy and mutual caring.
4. Develop guidelines and strategies for constructive conflict and effective communication.
5. Emphasize the couple's strengths and encourage positive, caring behaviors.

Experienced therapists will already be very familiar with these basic strategies and recognize both the value of Christensen's suggestions and when and how they can be applied successfully. It's encouraging for therapists already working in the field to have their intuition and experience reinforced by clinical research and empirical verification. For students of couple therapy and less experienced therapists, it is helpful to have a good understanding of strategies that work, when to use them, and in what contexts they work best. In addition to thoughts, feelings, and behaviors, we human beings also have physical sensations, vivid imaginations, and the ability to make decisions. Our ability to make conscious decisions is what makes us human beings. My golden retriever, for example, didn't have that ability. She was typically way too friendly and unable to exercise choice in the matter. I could appreciate her eagerness, but I usually had to apologize to visitors for her enthusiastic greetings. When she was threatened, she growled. Again, instincts prevailed, and she had little

---

9   Halweg, K., Grawe-Gerber, M., Baucom, D. (eds.). (2010). *Enhancing Couples*, p. 35.
10   The five central principles of Andrew Christensen's unified protocol are (1) provide a contextualized, dyadic, objective conceptualization of problems; (2) modify emotion-driven dysfunctional and destructive interactional behavior; (3) elicit avoided emotion-based private behavior; (4) foster productive communication; and (5) emphasize strengths and encourage positive behavior.

choice in the matter. When her perception of the threat went away, she returned to being obnoxiously friendly. She couldn't voluntarily moderate her emotions or her emotional responses. Humans can. The capacity for choice is one of the things that differentiate us from other mammals. And the capacity to make wise and loving choices is the fundamental goal of all forms of psychotherapy, and the heart of all successful relationships. When people are fighting like cats and dogs, they have fallen into instinctive, habitual, and defensive patterns of behavior. They've lost their most precious and distinctive human trait—the ability to make better choices.

The principles of change Christensen suggests target thoughts, behaviors, emotions, imagination, and choices. Change, it's important to remember, can occur by directing attention to any one of these areas. Helping couples to become aware of unrealistic expectations, for example, will help them let go of feelings of resentment or guilt. Making small efforts to treat each other differently will improve how they think and feel about their relationship. As they practice making better choices in talking to each other, it will be easier for them to feel like friends again. You will notice which areas of their relationship need attention first and suggest the best strategies for improvement.

Your tentative hypotheses will help you ask the right questions in order to zero in on what may be some of the underlying causes and unconscious motives holding your couple back from finding solutions. As in your previous session, you will ask how their week went and what they may have discussed since their last session. This will help you to determine whether to deal first with any current stressors or continue taking history, providing insight and education, and finish formulating and agreeing upon a treatment plan.

Sometimes therapy can proceed rapidly. Not all couples face serious problems, and some couples catch on quickly and make rapid progress. It's probably unlikely, but depending on the complexity of the issues involved, it may be possible to complete your therapy in just a few sessions. In fact, I recall a couple who needed help with their sexual relationship and got the help they needed after only one session. It wasn't too difficult. Gathering information from them I found out that they had six children under 12 years of age and no lock on their bedroom door. I suggested they buy a lock! Problem fixed! As far as I know they are living happily ever after. They were actually a pretty intelligent couple. They simply needed permission and encouragement to set better boundaries. They loved being a close family and wanted the kids to have access, but they also needed to be learn how to be okay with having some private time as a couple.

So, yes, some couple therapy can progress quickly, but it isn't the norm. Couples will sometimes ask me how long their therapy will take. Some years ago, I asked the contractor who was digging our future swimming pool the same question. "Depends," he said. "It shouldn't take very long unless we find water or rock." He found both. In a few cases, reasonable progress in therapy might be achieved in as few as six to eight weeks. But that's unusual. More commonly therapists find both water and rock. Some clients are easily flooded by difficult emotions. It takes time to build skills and develop strategies for containing or healing those emotions. For other couples, problems seem embedded in stone. Conflict patterns have become the hardpan of their relationship. Even jack-hammering through granite-hard attitudes and perceptions will hardly soften the ground. So how long will therapy take? As my contractor said, "it depends." Recall the advice I give to students: It depends on a couple's insightfulness, motivation, and maturity. Clients motivated to look at themselves and practice making better choices with their emotions and communication skills will typically make good progress.

Your Next Session

By your third appointment you have a fairly good idea of what's happening in the relationship. You have some tentative thoughts about your clients' personality styles—where they complement or challenge each other, how well they manage emotions and defenses, the types of problems and conflict patterns they struggle with, and how things might be improved. It's too soon to know for sure, but you will likely intuit the types of childhood conditioning they may have had, possible developmental wounds, attachment deficits, and emotional challenges that will surface in therapy.

This is your third session with Jim and Julie. You've asked how their week went and heard that things seem a little less tense at home. You'll explore what has improved and get a better idea of what emotions and behaviors may still need attention. You'll also continue taking history and developing your treatment plan— the quickest and most effective way to help. All treatment plans in therapy involve

- good definitions of the problem areas to be addressed;
- clearly identified, agreed-upon, and accessible goals;[11] and
- strategies for reaching those goals.

By the end of this session, you may have taken enough history and made sufficient observations to offer some insight into the nature of your couple's conflicts, how and why they may have developed, and what can be done to make things better. You'll be sure to consult with your couple about your thoughts and tentative plans. It's important that they have a voice and ownership of their therapy. The treatment plan requires clearly identifiable and *agreed-upon* goals. This means that they need to agree on the definition of the problems and the goals you want to reach. It might be good to suggest that each person make a list of what he or she would like to accomplish in therapy. Try to make the goals clear, simple, and possible to achieve. If the partners in the relationship are barely speaking to each other, or are easily provoked, encourage them to hold off on going over their issues with each other until they're in their therapy session. You will frame your therapy goals in ways that will make sense and have fewer sharp edges.

Not argue so much	Do more kind things for each other
Share tasks more equitably	Not withdraw as punishment
Have more fun	Spend more time together
Have more fulfilling sex life	Be better able to talk about feelings
Be more affectionate	Have a social life, make more friends
Have more of a spiritual life	Follow through with commitments
Be more honest and open	Keep the house more orderly
Agree on approaches to disciplining children	Not spend so much time on your cell phone

---

11   More rigorous treatment plans will call for goals that are also empirically verifiable.

Make better deals about managing
money, raising children, deciding
roles and responsibilities

After you've taken some time to agree on treatment goals, you will suggest strategies to reach those goals. Let's look again at Christensen's five fundamental strategies for couples and review some possible methods for reaching your goals. You will organize these strategies in ways that are tailored to improve your couple's relationship. Below are the strategies and the corresponding steps that I think make sense in accomplishing each one of your treatment goals.

Strategy 1: Develop a Clear Understanding of Each Partner's Contribution to Problems in the Relationship, Exposing the "Circular Causality" That Reinforces Ongoing Conflicts.

1. Identify differences in each partner's temperament and how those differences affect perception, decision-making, values, emotional expression, and how love is shared.
2. Acknowledge the differing influences of cultural and family conditioning.
3. Recognize differences in attachment styles and deficits and their influences in creating reciprocal wounding, reenactment, and subsequent patterns of conflict.

Strategy 2: Create Guidelines and Agreements for Containing Hurtful and Defensive Behaviors.

1. Be respectful of each other. Use words, not behaviors, to express negative feelings.
2. Watch your language. Never call your partner a bad name or refer to areas where they may be vulnerable. Never swear or use inflammatory language toward your partner. In some cases, this may constitute verbal or emotional abuse.
3. Contain your conflict. Agree on times to *avoid* arguing. Promise each other not to bring up sensitive topics after a certain time at night, in the car, on a date, or if you've been drinking. Bad timing, bad language, and poor discipline injure love and kill marriages.

Strategy 3: Access and Clarify Emotionally Charged Issues and Behaviors; Encourage Vulnerability, Empathy, and Mutual Caring.

1. Learn to identify your trigger issues, underlying emotions, and buried wounds.

2. Identify your defensive behaviors, such as attack or avoidance, and their root causes.
3. Practice self-disclosure, being more open and non-defensive with each other.

Strategy 4: Develop Guidelines and Strategies for Constructive Conflict and Effective Communication.

1. Set aside time for open and vulnerable discussions about your relationship.
2. Learn the skills of active listening and non-defensive communication.
3. Discipline yourself to use "time-outs" and constructive methods to resolve conflicts.

Strategy 5: Emphasize the Couple's Strengths and Encourage Positive, Caring Behaviors.

1. What have you survived or accomplished together? What do you like or appreciate about each other? In which areas do you work well together?
2. Find which behaviors would mean a great deal to your partner and do something daily.
3. Learn to affirm. That sounds trite, but kindness and simple compliments work wonders.

All couple therapy will likely include these basic strategies. Given the types of problems you see, the goals you want to reach, and the particulars of your couple's relationship, you and your couple will develop a plan for organizing and implementing the strategies that will work best in reaching their goals. Notice that each of the five strategies targets the three primary human traits of thinking, feeling, and behaviors.

Applying Christensen's Strategies

This is your fourth session with Jim and Julie and they seem to be doing better. Julie has noticed that Jim has made more of an effort to spend time with his son, Matt. They recently went to a ball game together and the dialogue between them, while minimal, is cordial. Julie has noticed that Jim seems less hostile and critical, and she has let him know that she appreciates the changes. What's interesting about Julie's report is that Jim has made these changes without any direct instruction from me. In their first session, I made a list of what they both wanted to work on. Jim wanted Julie to be more attentive to the house and firmer with the children's discipline.

Julie wanted Jim to have a better attitude and to be less hard on the kids. I also suggested, and they agreed, that it would be a good for them to learn and practice some communication and conflict management skills. I know, without asking, that right now they have a hard time spending time together, being affectionate, and that their sex life has suffered. I expect that this will all improve as they relate more successfully with each other. This has often been my experience; however, if their romantic life doesn't improve on its own, then that will also be included in our list of goals.

Obviously, my strategy here is to focus on the behaviors that are easier to change first. Frequently, small changes increase a couple's morale and motivation and things can improve more rapidly. While it feels good to enjoy a successful couple of weeks, I suspect that unless Jim and Julie learn and practice relationship skills, they may quickly find themselves back in their familiar rut. "Homeostasis" is a term that describes a tendency for a system to resist change.

Quoting again from *A General Theory of Love*:

> Because human beings remember with neurons, we are disposed to see more of what we have already seen, hear anew what we have heard most often, think just what we have always thought. Our minds are burdened by an informational inertia whose headlong course is not easy to slow.[12]

In *The Road Less Traveled*, Scott Peck described the same tendency when he discussed how difficult it is for human beings to "change the map of reality." Maturity, according to Peck, is the ability to respond successfully to the ongoing challenge of updating one's map. We will be discussing the concept of homeostasis again in the chapter on family systems. A couple conspires to create the story of their relationship. That story will not easily change. If, after a few weeks, your client couple decides that they have benefited from therapy and don't need to continue, try not to talk them out of that decision unless you see some serious problems that they haven't yet dealt with.

Give them your blessing but encourage them to come back for a "tune up" in a few weeks. They probably will. Motivation is very important for change and the motivation must come from them. It usually doesn't work to try to change their minds. You might suggest instead that they go to every other week. This will be easier on their budget and you can continue to give them the additional instruction and practice they need.

It's much more likely that you'll meet with a couple for at least three months and usually more, depending on the nature of their presenting problems. In the first few sessions you will focus on helping your couple understand why they're having such a hard time with their relationship. This will involve giving each person an opportunity to tell his or her own story. They can do this in your office because they can't do it at home. In most cases, they will be on better behavior in front of you and, if not, you can direct traffic. Speaking of which, you cannot do marriage counseling using a non-directive approach. You must be in control of the session. You can certainly be warm, encouraging, and polite. You can even allow your couple some time to fight in front of you. In fact, it's a good idea to listen in on how they argue—you'll quickly notice their defensive patterns and how their process breaks down. Clearly you can't allow the arguing to go more than a few minutes without losing control of the session. Your couple will quickly become frustrated with each other and with therapy if that happens. I've made that mistake a few times and had clients storm out of the session before I could help them take a time-out. Timing is important. You don't want to clamp down too soon or too often. Your couple needs to vent ... a bit. I'll interrupt if I think things are getting out of hand. "Let's take a time-out!" I'll stress (firmly if necessary). "Julie, please finish what you were saying. Jim, I'd like to have a better understanding of what Julie is feeling. then I would like to hear from you. But it works better if you both

---

12   Lewis, T., Amini, F., & Lannon, R. (2001). *A General Theory of Love*, p. 141.

give each other a turn." In your first one or two therapy sessions, you may feel like a traffic cop. You'll also function as an interpreter. Let's go back into our session with Jim and Julie to illustrate this.

Julie took her turn to be the speaker. I asked Jim to just listen and to try to hear the feelings that Julie was trying to express. "You're never home," she said. "You're always either at work or on the computer at home! We don't go out anymore. Obviously, I'm not important to you!" Jim just stared at her. "Julie," I said, "try this. Tell Jim you miss him." Julie teared up. "I do miss you," she said. Jim, obviously touched, replied, "I miss you too." "It works better," I suggested, "when you talk about your own feelings instead of criticizing the other person. You want to phrase what you're saying more as a confession and less like an indictment."

Much of what you're doing in therapy is helping people to hear each other—to listen more deeply into their own and their partner's story. One of the significant benefits of sitting in your office is that it's more likely that each person might actually hear what the other is saying. There is the likelihood that, without the typical defensive tug of war that characterizes their communication, they might be able to listen more objectively. To help this process along, you will do a lot of translating, clarifying, and reframing. You'll help your clients to hear feelings and not feel attacked.

You'll also help your clients to see possibilities. Recall that you are a professional listener. You've heard lots of stories—personally and professionally. Your training has prepared you to be able to understand the deeper dynamics alive inside of any given story. You can see potential and possibilities where your clients can't—at least, not yet. It's easier for you, sitting outside of your client's story, to see how the story started, the direction it's going, and what can be gained in terms of insight and growth. You also know what the story needs to be able to move forward to a favorable outcome.

When you begin helping your couple to understand the how and why of their story and where change can occur, you've changed hats again. You've gone from being a traffic cop, to a translator, and now to an educator. You will transition again shortly to become a trainer, then a coach, and end up, with luck, giving their graduation speech. You see what I mean about being directive. If you have trouble being sufficiently directive, couple therapy may not be right for you. You may wish to refer instead. The point is that your couple needs to feel that they are in the hands of a knowledgeable professional who can help them. You need to have faith that you can. You don't need to be arrogant or callous, just confident and firm with your advice and direction. Let' go back into session with Jim and Julie for more illustrations.

It's still their fourth session. As we heard above, they both report that things are better at home. You're happy to hear it, and when you ask them what has changed. They both state that the other seems more attentive and affectionate. Now that things are less tense at home, you suggest that it's a good time for them to learn how to have successful feeling talks, learn to make good deals, and manage conflict when it arises. You reassure them that conflict will occur at times but they will learn the skills to deal with it more successfully, understand why it occurs, and how to learn and grow from conflict. You're especially pleased that Jim seems to be on board with the communication training. You wondered, after their first session, if he would be willing to be vulnerable and talk about some of the things that he was feeling. It turns out he can. This is good news, especially since so many males and some females have a difficult time understanding the purpose of a "feeling talk." You put on your teacher's hat and go to work explaining why feeling talks are important and how to have them successfully. After a brief lecture (see the communication guidelines in the appendix) you announce that you will now be shifting from lecture to lab. That means that you will be asking your client couple to turn and face each other. You'll suggest that one of them be the speaker and the other the listener; you ask them to practice the guidelines that you've just taught them. This is a pivotal point in therapy, and you need to be careful when you suggest it. If the motivation and maturity is sufficient, and if they're not in the midst of a heated argument, you can suggest that they will be doing two things at once—they will be discussing content issues while practicing process.

As I've stated above, helping them learn *process* is ultimately more valuable than spending time helping them to negotiate *content*. Sometimes couples catch on quickly and do a good job of using their "speaker–listener" skills within the first two or three sessions. Other couples may take months and still be challenged not to interrupt, get defensive, and become argumentative. The steps to good communication—taking turns, not interrupting, discussing one's own feelings instead of attacking, and giving feedback to the speaker that his or her message has gotten across—are very easy to understand and very difficult to apply. It's like overlaying a thin set of guidelines on top of potentially explosive emotions. It takes lots of practice. This is why I think Andrew Christensen is right when he argues with Gottman and observes that communication training can be very effective when it is taught skillfully, learned thoroughly, and practiced repeatedly. As soon as you feel your client couple is ready, shift from lecture to lab.

Jim and Julie are facing each other. Julie has "confessed" to missing Jim. Her vulnerability is moving. It's Jim's turn to give his wife feedback. He does a good job. He makes a small, common mistake by saying "I miss you too." Technically he shouldn't be the speaker until he has given her feedback about what he's heard. But in this context it's what she needs to hear and you'll let it go. Jim doesn't know yet that the best feedback he can give Julie is to simply say, "I get that my being absent so much has made you sad, and you miss me." "I really do," Julie would probably say. I realize that saying "thanks for listening" sounds weird and too formal. Be sure to give your couple permission to laugh about having to say that when they're doing a feeling talk, but have them practice it anyway. It's hard to be a good listener. When Kathe and I are having a feeling talk, we usually say that to each other, not because we're therapists but because it works to let the other person know that you appreciate the time and effort they took to give you their full attention. It's also a shorthand way of saying, "I'm done. Now you can be the speaker." If saying "thanks for listening" sounds too formal and foreign, suggest that your couple simply say "I'm done." Also explain that a "feeling talk" *will* seem formal and foreign. It's not how people usually talk to each other. Thank goodness.

A feeling talk is a special time for following specific guidelines intended to help people feel safe enough to be vulnerable. It is necessarily formal. You're taking your time, going slowing and carefully through a potential minefield of explosive emotions. You take turns, listen, give feedback, and move over the emotional terrain carefully enough to truly hear and feel heard. When a feeling talk is done successfully, partners are metaphorically taking their clothes off and standing naked in front of each other. They touch each other's souls. It can be just as enjoyable and fulfilling as lovemaking. In fact, having regular success with the depth and tenderness of this level of communication will certainly enhance a couple's physical lovemaking. When I teach classes on sexuality, I frequently state that the majority of problems couples experience with sex are, in actuality, problems with emotional intimacy. Typically, when couples can make love emotionally, things work much better physically.

Now it's Jim's turn to be the speaker. You know what he's likely to say. But he surprises you a bit with his ability to be vulnerable as well. "I feel a lot of pressure," he says, "mostly about finances. I feel pressure to do a good job at work and, frankly, I feel a lot of pressure at home. I want to be a good husband and father. Sometimes I feel that everything is on my shoulders and I guess I get kind of resentful." "I understand," Julie replies. "I can see that you could feel pressured and resentful." She wants to say more, such as, "why do you need to work such long hours, and why do you have to be such a perfectionist about everything!" But, luckily, she remembers that it's not her turn. "You're a hard worker," she says, "we appreciate you!" "Thanks for listening," Jim says and genuinely means it. It's been far too long since he felt appreciated.

"Great job," I can say—and truly mean it. I'm happy that they've had a successful feeling talk. And before they have a chance to ask me the usual question, "where do we go from here?" I remind them that having your feelings heard and feeling cared about is huge. In some marriages, it's non-existent. When conflict can't be resolved it's typically because partners don't believe that their feelings and perspective have been heard and valued. Once a person feels truly understood and cared about, he or she is more motivated to work with the other person to find a deal that they can both live with.

Julie could show Jim more appreciation, and she also could be more affectionate. I'll ask them if their feeling talk in my office has translated into improvements at home. I like when change happens organically instead of my prescribing it. It's not unusual for me to give couples the standard assignment of writing out things they appreciate about the other and things they would like to see improved. In fact, I will occasionally recommend marital checklists of one type or another.

A feeling talk is a special type of communication. It's strictly about feelings, not solving problems. If a feeling talk drifts towards problem-solving, a couple will likely miss the opportunity to go very deep and really hear what's at stake for each other. You'll tell your couple that much of the time they'll want to wait a bit, maybe a day or so, to put some time between a feeling talk and problem-solving. I would like to think that based on their feeling talk, Jim and Julie have a pretty good idea of what they need to focus on at home. Therapists frequently want to give homework to couples. I'm no exception. In this case, however, I think I'll wait. I hope that it's as clear to them as it is to me that Jim needs to be more attentive and affectionate to Julie and the kids. Julie could show Jim more appreciation and also be more affectionate. I'm hoping that these behaviors will arise organically—that the changes come from them, rather than my having to prescribe them.

There are some homework assignments, however, that I typically do prescribe. The obvious assignment that many therapists use is for the couple to write out the things that they appreciate about each other and the things they would like the other to work on. For this assignment, I'll ask Jim and Julie to take a Marital Checklist. I've used this checklist for many years and included it in the appendix for your use. I'll ask the couple to take the checklist to fill out at home, and I'll give them a bit of instruction while they're still in the office. I'll instruct Jim, for example, to check the behaviors he would like Julie to focus more attention on and, also, to place an "x" next to what he thinks Julie is checking on her list. I'll have Julie do the same thing. This way, when they bring in their checklists, I'll be able to see what improvements each person is asking for from the other as well as whether the information is getting through (if Julie's x's correspond to Jim's checks, and vice versa).

In situations like this it's essential that you first instruct your couple on how to have successful feeling talks. Both partners need to hear that the other respects their values and is willing to work to find a common approach—that their feelings matter. Once that's accomplished, they will be better able to work together as a team instead of feeling like opponents. So both Jim and Julie have had their feeling talk about what's at stake for each of them in their approach to disciplining Matt. I look at Jim and ask him what he would like to do differently. I let Julie know that I will be asking her the same question next. I remind them that I'm not asking what they want the other person to do but what each of them, individually, plan to work on. So far, Jim and Julie have been fairly mature and respectful of each other so I'm pretty sure that we can move the discussion toward problem-solving.

There are two main ways to solve problems: internal and external. Internal problem-solving requires two people finding something they can both agree to. External problem-solving is about one partner getting his or her way this time and the other partner next time. Kathe and I go out for lunch together on Wednesday afternoons. We set that time to see each other because much of the rest of week is spent seeing clients. Next week it will be Kathe's turn to choose which restaurant we go to. That's an easy external solution. She's better at handling finances than I am—another good external solution. And I find myself doing most of the yard work. You get the idea.

It's possible for parents to take turns disciplining their children; just like they took turns getting up to comfort their newborn at night. It's possible, but unfortunately, it's not very realistic. Ideally, parents agree on expectations and consequences for the kids. Favorable consequences typically work best to positively reinforce good behavior. Taking away a privilege can be used to extinguish bad behavior. The expectations and consequences are agreed upon and posted somewhere so that it's clear to everyone what needs to happen, in what time frame, and what consequence, positive or negative, will follow. I've included a parenting plan in the appendix to suggest a strategy for parents to (literally) be on the same page with each other regarding discipline. The parenting plan invites parents to work together to assign tasks, monitor attitudes, check on academic performance, and agree on reasonable positive and negative consequences consistently applied by both parents.

Jim and Julie have transitioned from their feeling talk and begun to do some problem-solving. I'm happy that I don't have to spell it out for them. Jim has answered my question about what he plans to work on at home. He says that he plans to do something with Matt that Matt will enjoy. He will also trust Julie to monitor both children's homework and household chores and work with her to develop a list of expectations and consequences for the kids. He also said that he will try to be in a better mood at home and be more affectionate. Julie said that she plans to be more attentive to the kid's behavior; that she will monitor their chores and homework and be more careful about her spending.

This is a good beginning for this couple and a good place to end the session. We've been talking for about 45 minutes, and I want to end on a positive note. So I'll try to defer any last-minute tension by announcing that, with the time remaining, I'd like to summarize what we've discussed in this session. I try to end the session positively, sending them home in a good place. Good luck with that.

I'll be clear with couples that I don't want them to bring up any difficult topics or emotions just before the end of the session. That's easier said than done. With highly conflicted couples, I typically recommend that, to keep the peace at home, they make notes to themselves of anything that comes up during the week that is upsetting and bring what they've written to our next session. Write things out instead of bringing things up ... at least for this week. "Later," I say, "I will give you the opposite advice. Once you've learned how to talk things out successfully, I will encourage you to have your feeling talks at home."

I summarize, for Jim and Julie, the progress they've made in therapy. I congratulate them on a successful feeling talk and being able to develop a plan for working together as co-parents. I'm fully aware that this won't be the end of their therapy. There has been a lot of hurt in this family.

Matt may not respond quickly, or at all, to his father's attempts to get closer to him. Julie is well-intentioned but will have a hard time being as strict with the kids as Jim expects. There will be more arguing and more hurt feelings. Jim and Julie haven't spent nearly enough time practicing their speaker–listener skills or learning how to turn an argument around. They don't yet fully trust each other, and the pull of their familiar ways of operating will threaten to distance them again.

In conclusion, I'll warn them they had one good session but there is still much to learn and practice and I'm happy that they are making this commitment to continue to work on their relationship.

"Next week, we'll continue to practice your skills," I'll say, "and follow up on your individual work. Don't forget to fill out your marriage checklist, and I hope you have a good week. See you next time."

Questions for Discussion

1. As a therapist, will it be more likely that you will be directive or non-directive?
2. In what situations are you likely to be less directive or more directive?
3. What makes it hard for you to be directive?
4. What makes it hard for you to be non-directive?
5. What do you think are the top three goals to work toward in couple therapy?

CHAPTER THIRTEEN

Family Stories

CHAPTER SUMMARY AND LEARNING OBJECTIVE

I said this about couples, but it's also true for families: they are like noses. We all have one. They're all different and they're all alike. This chapter defines and describes families. While families are unique, they all have dynamics in common such as structure, a process of conveying information and expectation, family roles, family rules, and family rituals, to name a few. It's important for therapists to understand the interplay of these diverse dynamics and how they function to maintain stability and homeostasis. It's also important to recognize the systemic nature of family functioning and how changing one aspect of that functioning affects the rest of the system. Therapy can address the family's structure, process, roles, and rules as an initial approach to creating change. There are diverse strategies for creating change in families with the goal of enabling healthier choices.

The learning objective for this chapter is to be able to define the term "family" and to explain the commonalities and systemic nature of family functioning.

All therapy is family therapy. Does that seem like an exaggeration? When you consider the significant influence families have on your clients' development and current functioning, their family *is* in your office whether you see them or not. It's true that family therapy is a specialized type of therapy in which all or most of the family members are physically present in your office. But it's very important to have a good understanding of family systems and the various approaches and skills needed to help families, whether you have one or all of the family members present.

Families influence how we behave socially and in significant relationships, how we view the world, what we value, and even how our brain develops. In *The Developing Mind*, Dan Siegel says that "caregivers are the architects of the way in which experience influences the unfolding of genetically preprogrammed but experience-dependent brain development. Genetic potential is expressed within the setting of social experiences" (p. 85). Families nurture us and wound us. Families teach us about love and shame, about guilt and grace, and, in a very real sense, however distant we may be and whether we like it or not, our family is always present with us.

I have two goals in writing this section of the book on narrative systems in families. The first goal is to help you become better acquainted with how your own family of origin has influenced your development. This will help you with the second goal which is to become more knowledgeable about family functioning in general and how to work successfully with families in therapy. To achieve these goals, I will briefly discuss the various dynamics that all families share and a variety of therapeutic approaches for helping families heal and grow. In addition, I will suggest some exercises to help you apply these dynamics to better understand your own family. Next, I will suggest a model that places many of the techniques of family therapy in a visual structure that will help you determine which therapeutic approach will likely work best with a given type of family problem.

Families Defined

There are many ways to define the word "family." I like Wikipedia's definition: "a group of people affiliated by consanguinity (blood relation), affinity, or co-residence." That seems to be adequately simple and appropriately broad. It means that "Aunt" Martha, who is no relation at all and lives alone but is always invited to special family occasions, is "related" by affiliation. Her title of Aunt or Auntie is a favorite in many cultures around the world because it signifies a special kind of relationship. It may be that when you invite all the members of your client family into therapy, it will be important to include Aunt Martha or Uncle Bob or anyone else who has been considered a "family member."

Family Dynamics

All family stories share elements in common. There is *structure*—how families operate, how power is distributed, and how things get done. Families have *process*—the way in which information is conveyed. Families have *history*—roots and resources. And whether they realize it or not, families have *goals* and direction. Families are healthy when the family structure supports the goals of the family and the growth and well-being of individual members, and when communication is clear, consistent, and respectful. The family's structure reveals the *roles* and responsibilities of family members. Process is governed by family *rules*—the spoken and unspoken directives that govern what individuals may or may not do. A family's history can provide the emotional *resources* of meaning and continuity and contribute to a family's *reality*—its goals and openness to the future. Families share rituals. The word *ritual* may have its roots in the word for *river*. Rituals flow through the lifespan of a family, conveying continuity and celebrating developmental milestones. The diagram below will help you see the connection and interaction of these family dynamics. I alliterated the key internal workings of the family system to make them easier to remember.

PROCESS

Rules
(clear or ambiguous)

HISTORY	Resources	Rituals	Reality	GOALS
	(energizing or enervating)	*(meaningful or empty)*	*(open or closed)*	

Roles
(fair or unfair)

STRUCTURE

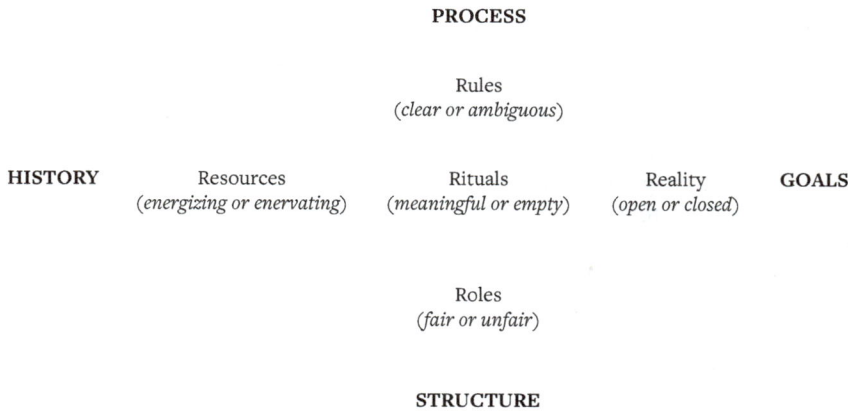

FIG. 13-1 How Families Function

Family Stressors

All families face two broad categories of stressors: *vertical* and *horizontal*. Horizontal stressors consist of both the normal developmental challenges of life as well as extraordinary events that cause more traumatic types of stress. Perhaps a family begins with two people deciding to become a couple. That has some built-in stresses. Children may enter the picture—more stress. Financial challenges, relocation, late hours, in-laws, illness, education, job changes, divorce, etc.—life is full of stresses on families. Vertical stressors consist of how successfully or unsuccessfully a family deals with its horizontal stressors. Vertical stressors often reveal the level of maturity, resourcefulness, and cooperation in a family system. And if the vertical skills and resources are not up to the horizontal challenges, you may get a phone call.

Family Systems

John Bradshaw's books and seminars have been popular for the past three decades. In his seminars, Bradshaw will often hold up a mobile with one hand and gently touch one portion of the mobile with the other. Bradshaw is showing us that nudging one element of a system will affect the entire system. So it is with families. In the past five decades, as more and more people opened to the idea of family counseling, it has become increasingly clear to therapists that individual clients would frequently present with symptoms that resulted directly from dysfunctional family systems. In addition, when facing significant, or even normal, life stressors, enlightened families are realizing that the whole family needs the guidance and stabilizing influence of an "outside" person. I place the word "outside" in quotes because one of the fundamental tenants of family therapy is that once a family comes in for therapy, the therapist becomes part of the system. This is the *mobile effect*, and the addition of a therapist to the system may help a family get through tough times.

Realizing an obvious need, pioneers in family therapy developed a host of strategies and techniques for treating the whole family. In general, these techniques focus on the family's structure, the family's process, and the family's most immediate problem. Addressing any one of these areas will typically unbalance the family's *homeostasis* and create a climate where improvement is possible. Two important terms in the language of family systems are "unbalancing" and "homeostasis." Homeostasis is the tendency for systems to remain resistant to change. That can be especially true for family systems. When our three grown daughters panic at the suggestion that we change a time-honored holiday tradition, we know that homeostasis has come home for the holidays.

An effort to introduce a new tradition or discard an old one will "unbalance" the homeostasis. Unbalancing can be a good thing when it comes to stimulating the growth of individuals or families, but it's often a very unpopular idea in practice. In some families, unbalancing homeostasis is not only unpopular but also impossible. One way to measure the health of a family is to notice the family's openness to change. Openness to change is one of the hallmarks of mature functioning. A mature person is typically open to new information and changing behaviors. He or she can manage impulses and moderate emotions so that they do not significantly impair rational decision-making. Immature people cannot. Murray Bowen, one of the early family therapists, has a word for this kind of mature functioning. He called it "differentiation."

Family Differentiation, Motivation, and Openness to Change

The methods you use to help a family with their problems will typically depend on the three qualities above—the family's level of differentiation, their motivation, and their openness to change. Bowen observed that when people get married, it's usually to a person with a similar level of differentiation. It makes sense that people who are mature enough to be open to change and can adequately manage their emotions would not be romantically interested in people who weren't. It also makes sense that these people would be more likely to raise their children to have similar values. The "nuclear family emotional system" is the result. That's Bowen's phrase for the level of emotional maturity characteristic of any given family. This continuum suggests how successfully a family will deal with horizontal stressors as well as the likelihood that they would benefit from family therapy. But the family's level of differentiation is only one factor in predicting a successful outcome to family therapy. Just as important is the family's openness to change and their motivation to work together for growth.

Motivation is a simple concept to grasp, but understanding why a family is motivated to begin therapy, what they're motivated to achieve, and how to keep them motivated can be pretty complex. Openness to change is also a complex topic. It requires keeping an open mind and a willingness to explore new ideas and ways of improving. I think that most people would agree with that concept but find it hard to apply. Scott Peck (as noted previously) reflected on this point in the *Road Less Traveled* when he commented on how difficult it is for people to "change their map of reality." So, again, when it comes to working with families, the methods you choose will largely depend on the family's level of differentiation, motivation, and openness to change.

Keep in mind that family systems are very complex, and you may need to be flexible and adapt your approach as therapy progresses.

Family Therapy, Eight Approaches

It won't take you very long to assess your client family's motivation, differentiation, etc. You'll determine the presenting problem, your client family's resources and work areas, and you'll begin to think about the best way to help them. Below are the eight most important therapeutic approaches that you'll want to be familiar with. They're categorized according to the approaches that deal primarily with *structure*, with *process*, or with the *presenting problem*. Of course, you'll find overlapping characteristics in all of these methods. It's best to think about these therapeutic methods on a continuum that emphasizes process or structure on one end of the continuum and dealing directly with the family's presenting problem on the opposite end. Below is a brief description of the eight approaches.

Experiential Family Therapy

Experiential family therapy focuses on *process*. Virginia Satir and Carl Whitaker were both advocates of helping client families become more aware of their emotions, more successful in the expression of their emotions, and more skilled in clear and direct communication. Change and growth occur as family members *experience* each other through mutual sharing.

Narrative Family Therapy

Narrative family therapy is also a *process-oriented* approach with an emphasis on the family's "reality"—how family members perceive themselves, their relationships, and their challenges. The goal of narrative family therapy is to help family members develop a healthier *story*, consisting of a more positive outlook, the ability to reframe problems, and to become more open to discover new insights for finding creative solutions. A useful intervention would be to explore the family's history and values in order to find key elements in the storyline of the family.

Psychodynamic and Transgenerational Family Therapy

Psychodynamic and transgenerational family therapy could be considered a type of *process-oriented* therapy in the sense that these approaches focus on the processes by which ways of seeing and being in the world are passed on from generation to generation. Alfred Adler and, later, Murray Bowen focused on understanding the importance of social and family conditioning on the emotional and behavioral health of individuals. As in narrative therapy, these approaches rely on insight and direct experience to produce change. A useful intervention would be for the family to work together to create a family genogram.

Cognitive-Behavioral Family Therapy

Cognitive-behavioral family therapy views the family's *process* from classic CBT constructs of those automatic thoughts and core beliefs that affect how problems are envisioned and approached. In CBFT, the therapist is very directive in educating, confronting, and exposing emotions, beliefs, and behaviors that keep the family stuck. A useful intervention for this family would be to discuss and practice ways in which to positively reframe how each family member views the family as a whole and family members individually.

Structural Family Therapy

Structural family therapy, as the title suggests, focuses on the family *structure*, the ways a family organizes itself, the roles and rituals that create systems and subsystems, and the types of boundaries that functionally or dysfunctionally maintain family homeostasis. Using various techniques and homework, the therapist helps the family identify the dysfunctional interaction patterns and unbalances the existing system to create healthier boundaries and subsystems. An "unbalancing" structural intervention may be as simple as directing the parents to sit closer together, not separated by a child or children in the therapy session.

Strategic Family Therapy

Strategic family therapy is on the side of the continuum that focuses more directly on dealing with the family's *presenting problem*. The therapy sessions involve developing a clear idea of the problems the family is facing, formulating plans to address these problems, and assigning homework to create both first- and second-order change. As in CBFT, the therapist is directive and functions to guide the family to find solutions. One interesting spin on SFT is the "systemic" Milan school which frequently uses a therapy team hidden behind a one-way mirror. The team consults and advises in the therapy. The Milan method also features "paradoxical prescriptions" that *assign* the "apparent" problem in order to expose the actual problems in the family system.

Solution-Focused Family Therapy

Solution-focused family therapy is typically brief and very *problem* (solution)-*focused*. The therapist attempts to move the family away from assigning blame and discussing the origins of the problem to focusing on solutions. The therapist digs into the family's story, finds resources, explores exceptions to the family's perceived problems, and helps the family envision their preferred future. The emphasis is on taking small, immediate steps toward motivating family members to make progress in creating change.

An Integrative Approach

The first step in developing an integrative approach to doing family therapy is to thoroughly understand how family systems operate—to understand concepts such as homeostasis, circular causality, second-order change, boundaries, structure, identified patient, and so forth. You need to be fluent in the language of family systems. Second, it's important to thoroughly understand the goals and methods of the traditional approaches described above. Each approach offers important insights into families and how family members affect and are affected by their family systems. Each approach offers valuable therapeutic methods that work. The third step is to assess your client family, to get to know their structure, process, openness to change, and levels of maturity and motivation. As an illustration of an integrative approach, here are some suggestions for conducting your first family session and what to look for in making an initial assessment. You'll notice examples from many of the therapy approaches listed above. You and your client family will determine what order works best.

In preparation for seeing a family, you may wish to review Bowen's Differentiation of Self Scale. I included a modified version in the appendix. Having this scale in mind will help you make a good guess about your client family's level of maturity. In greeting your family in the waiting room, be sure to say hello and shake hands with *each* family member, adult or child.

1. Get to know your family and help them relax. Use circular questioning to get basic information such as ages and grade levels of children, what people like and would change about their family, their family rules and rituals, and favorite stories. What does this family consider as their strengths?
2. Notice where people are sitting in your office and invite the family to question why they chose the seats they did. You may decide to make a "structural" intervention and invite people to sit in different spots. Notice any resistance and comments.
3. Get the family members' ideas about why they are in therapy and what problems they want to fix. Have the family decide what problems to work on first. How motivated do they seem—how open to change?
4. Notice if someone may be acting out or perceived by others in the family as being the problem. (The identified patient (IP) is the person that family members agree is the one causing problems in the family. Realistically, the IP may well be the healthiest member of a dysfunctional family. The "acting out" is a form of expressing the need for change.)
5. Summarize this initial session, give them a "preview of coming attractions" (what to expect from therapy), and be positive about their family's ability to face challenges, meet goals, and solve problems.

The diagram in the next chapter will help guide you to consider what approach(s) to begin with. Adjust your approach or apply techniques from other approaches based on your client family's apparent level of differentiation, motivation, openness, and resourcefulness.

Questions for Discussion

1. How would you characterize your nuclear family's story?
2. How would you characterize the past history of your family?
3. How would you characterize your mother's role in her family growing up?
4. How would you characterize your father's role in his family growing up?
5. How would you characterize your family's values?
6. What do you think are important values for all families?

CHAPTER FOURTEEN

Matching Your Therapeutic Approach to the Family

CHAPTER SUMMARY AND LEARNING OBJECTIVE

Selecting the best therapeutic approach to treat a family can be very confusing. Over the years, family therapists have developed seven major treatment approaches: structural, strategic, experiential, psychodynamic, cognitive, narrative, and solution-focused. One can also use an *integrative* approach, intelligently combining interventions from various treatment approaches.

Key factors for determining which approaches and interventions to use are the level of differentiation of a family, their commitment to change, their openness to alternative perspectives and choices, and the resources available to the family. This chapter includes a diagram placing the major components of family functioning in a circle alongside the key factors mentioned above. Using this diagram, the therapist can more easily determine which type of family therapy might work best with any given family. The chapter describes each therapeutic approach in detail, along with the terms used to describe family functioning, level of differentiation, motivation, openness to change, resources, and so forth.

The learning objective for this chapter is to describe the key factors in determining which of the major approaches to use in treating families and to provide a rationale for selecting a particular treatment approach.

Finding the Best Approach to Treating Your Client Family

On the following page, I provide a template for assessing the strengths and weaknesses of your client family. You determine the best approach to treatment based on four criteria: the family's *level of differentiation*, their level of *motivation*, their *history*, and their *goals*. As stated above, a family's differentiation describes the level of mature or immature family functioning. A high level of differentiation for a family, as for an individual, is the ability to make wise decisions in the midst of difficult emotions. Mature individuals can do that fairly consistently. Clearly, a family needs to be motivated to improve, regardless of the difficulty involved. A high level of motivation is a good predictor of success. The family history can be an asset and a resource if the family members can draw on traditions of close connections and working together to find solutions to family challenges. An example may be, "We are a close-knit family that has overcome adversity."

Whether stated or not, all families have goals. Sometimes the goal is to keep things, as much as possible, the way they are. Sometimes the goals are for education, or employment, or marriage and children. For a family to be successful in therapy, you hope to see that the family is open to change—that they have an *open reality*. An open reality means that the family is capable of looking at things with an open mind. They're not encrusted in philosophies about how people should be, how families should be, how the world should be.

Higher levels of differentiation are usually an indication that your client family is able to understand the value of looking at their *process*—how they communicate with each other. They may not need much encouragement or instruction to experience each other in different ways, and they can readily learn to convey information clearly, directly, and respectfully. These families can be open to interpreting their experiences in better ways, to write different stories, and to create healthier outcomes. In addition, if your client family is highly motivated, an *experiential* or *narrative* approach or combination of each may be the most efficient and effective methods.

Other process-oriented approaches such as *psychodynamic* or *transgenerational* also require fairly high levels of differentiation. These families are able to be open to new insights about how family members have been shaped by childhood conditioning and experiences and how that conditioning affects their style and expectations of interpersonal relationships.

Relational patterns develop out of those interpersonal relationships, forming systems and subsystems that benefit or impair healthy family functioning. These approaches may help families who need the additional motivation provided by insight and understanding into why they experience the challenges they do and how best to meet those challenges.

Cognitive-behavioral therapy emphasizes both insight and rehearsal. Because this approach requires learning and practicing skills, it may not be the most efficient approach, but it's a good way to help families create lasting change. Insight and motivation develop as, over time, family members see results and become practiced at seeing and reacting to problems more effectively. This may be the best approach to use with families who will benefit from concrete goals, instruction, encouragement, and homework.

Structural and *strategic* approaches work well with families that may not be as motivated to change. These families are focusing on immediate *problems* and are more interested in solutions than insight. Problems may result from unhealthy patterns of interacting and from how power is shared, used, or abused. The goal of therapy with these families is to directly confront, disturb, or unbalance the dysfunctional interactions and patterns of power so that healthier patterns can emerge.

Solution-focused therapy is similarly oriented to fixing problems. The family's energy and imagination are directed toward working together to explore possible solutions. In the process of focusing on the problem, the family discovers (with the help of the therapist) that they are able to work together. This method can also be an effective approach with families that may not be as motivated to participate in long-term, insight-oriented therapy.

Copy this page and use it to assess the best therapeutic approach for your family.

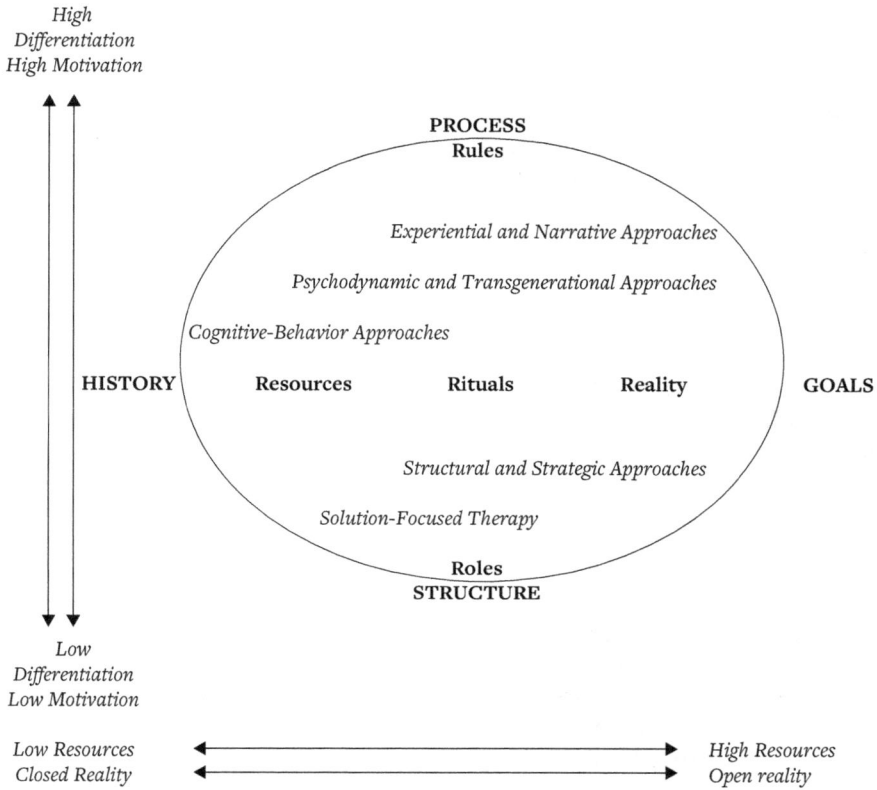

High
Differentiation
High Motivation

PROCESS
Rules

Experiential and Narrative Approaches

Psychodynamic and Transgenerational Approaches

Cognitive-Behavior Approaches

HISTORY   **Resources**   **Rituals**   **Reality**   **GOALS**

Structural and Strategic Approaches

Solution-Focused Therapy

Roles
STRUCTURE

Low
Differentiation
Low Motivation

Low Resources   *High Resources*
Closed Reality   *Open reality*

Family Rules:

Family Roles:

Family Rituals:

Family Resources:

Family Reality:

It's possible to successfully employ one of these approaches in its pure theoretical format. It's more likely that you'll find yourself borrowing ideas and methods from various approaches as therapy evolves, as you get to know your client family's strengths and work areas, and as problem areas migrate from process to structure, and so forth. Over time, you'll become more experienced at reading families and the challenges they face, and you will have greater facility with finding the quickest and most durable methods to help them. This is one of the more enjoyable and engaging aspects of working within a family systems framework.

Questions for Discussion and Exercises

The goal of this section is to help you become even more familiar with the workings of a family system—in this case, your own family system. As a student of marriage and family therapy at California Lutheran University in 1983, I was asked to write a paper entitled "The Differentiation of Myself from My Family of Origin." That was the first time I began to look seriously and, in some respects, critically at the family I grew up in. I investigated the family rules that operated in my home, the roles that guided our interactions together, and the family myths and rituals that gave us a sense of identity and continuity. MFT students have been asked to write similar papers ever since. It can certainly be an eye-opening, if not alarming, experience—but valuable in either case. The value is multifaceted. It will help you to know yourself better. That's important for many reasons, not the least of which is that, as a therapist, it's essential to know where you leave off and someone else begins. Your family experience will not necessarily be identical to their experience; and the family rules that continue to guide you may be completely foreign to them. Another goal of this exercise is to give you insight into your own experience of "differentiation." How well do you differentiate thoughts, feelings, and choices from your family of origin, and how does your level of differentiation help or hinder your important relationships? Another unavoidable goal is to help you become more empathic with the emotional challenges your clients face when they look at their own families of origin. As I stated above, this process will be informative; it may also be unsettling. Be honest in your inquiry but also exercise good self-care. Pace yourself and find emotional support if you need to. Here are four additional exercises that will be useful for you personally as well as for your clients.

Exercise #1: Differentiation

In the appendix of this workbook you'll find Murray Bowen's Modified Differentiation of Self Scale. No one will see the results of this test, so be honest with yourself and see where you come out in your level of internal and external differentiation. It will be interesting to consider your parents' level of differentiation, the family rules they inherited that promoted or discouraged their own differentiation, and what rules were handed down to you. It may also be useful to consider the effects of your own degree of differentiation on the types of romantic relationships you've experienced.

Exercise #2: Family Rules

A family rule is an explicit (overt, verbalized) or implicit (covert, non-verbalized) directive regarding expectations of behaviors, emotions, attitudes, and even thoughts and opinions. Family rules along with family rituals (celebrating special events and occasions) and family myths (our family is a _____ family) combine to inform our inner scripts or narratives—the stories we tell ourselves about who we are and what is correct and expected. The family rules we learn growing up can continue to influence every aspect of our life: morality, relationships, self-care, health, spirituality, sexuality, and so forth. A good way to get in touch with some of these family rules is to write out all of the rules that you are aware of (many of them were unspoken). Write out Dad's rules and Mom's rules. Notice if the rules were similar or competitive. What rules have you kept over the years? What rules have you reacted against or modified? What rules have you made for yourself? Here are some typical categories to explore: spending money, school grades, expressing feelings, health issues, religious involvement, acceptable dinner conversation, neatness, politics, responsibilities, etc. You or your clients may have grown up not knowing a father or mother. In some of these cases, a rule may be, "Don't expect me to be in your life." In other cases, where the absence was unavoidable, a rule might be, "Don't expect life to be fair." You get the idea. Write out as many of these spoken and unspoken rules as you can think of. If you are willing and open, this will take some time. Keep a notebook handy as you recall more examples. You should end up with at least three to four pages of Dad's rules, Mom's rules, and your own rules.

Exercise #3: Family Roles

Alfred Adler was one of the first theorists to appreciate that family members often took on specific roles contributing to a "family constellation." He was particularly interested in the effect that birth order has in cultivating these roles. One often finds both functional and dysfunctional roles among family members. Roles help to distribute the workload and responsibilities of living or working together. When the roles and responsibilities are clearly defined and fair, the family benefits. It is very likely, however, that the family sitting in your office is there because of problems with roles. The parenting is inequitable, for example. The workload is not divided fairly. Power is misused. A child is acting out the role of the "attention seeker," the "oppositional teenager," the "bookish loner," the "addict." It's important to understand how roles can be beneficial as well as how roles can be used to manage or maintain family dysfunction. What were some of the roles operating in your family of origin? In what ways did these roles support a healthy or unhealthy family life?

Exercise #4: Family Rituals

Family rituals have symbolic meaning for the family. Birthdays, holidays, coming-of-age celebrations, family nights, family meals, and family vacations are some of the many recurring events that give meaning and continuity to family life and, ideally, express value and appreciation to family members. Many family traditions and rituals have cultural and religious roots that are adopted and modified and given special meaning. These rituals create contexts in which family history and traditions may be recalled and kept alive for future generations. They may also be sources of conflict within and between families. In one sense all families are "cross-cultural"; that is, every family has its own way of celebrating events that may differ significantly from other families within similar cultural and religious contexts.

Where the newly married couple decides to spend the holidays, for example, may be another measure of the flexibility and maturity of their respective families. In this exercise, I would like you to recall some of the important family rituals you experienced growing up—the ones you looked forward to and the ones you didn't. What meaning and significance did these rituals convey? You may recall some conflicts created by these rituals. You may also reflect on the difference between a meaningful ritual and an empty ritualization—a repeated event devoid of the enjoyment and meaning that it ought to have. What were some of your family rituals?

Exercise #5: Genogram

A genogram is a pictorial display of a person's family tree showing repetitive patterns of behavior. Genograms help you visualize the traits and tendencies passed down from generation to generation. Your family process paper should include your family genogram going back to your grandparents at least. There are ample resources online to create your genogram. The experience you gain in developing your own genogram as well as the process you will undertake in writing out your own family rules, roles, and rituals will be extremely useful. In the process of unearthing issues and emotions you may not have been aware of you'll become more sensitive to the issues and emotions your clients may experience and you will be better able to differentiate your own issues from your clients' issues.

CHAPTER FIFTEEN

Thoughts on Therapy and Culture

CHAPTER SUMMARY AND LEARNING OBJECTIVE

This chapter summarizes what I believe about doing effective therapy. Therapists have their own individual style. What matters most is not necessarily your treatment plan but your genuine regard for your client. Warmth, curiosity, and encouragement, added to your training and experience, will create a context where change and healing can happen. The quality of attunement is vital to create an environment of trust and transformation. You are a professional listener, and you hear your client's story against the myriad of human stories you've learned in your training. You listen with your *head* to gain understanding. You listen with your *heart* to experience empathy and to create a connection. You listen with your *spirit* to confer value to an "other" human being. Few people have the opportunity to be asked "What is it like to be you?" This is the wonderful opportunity and challenge you have as a psychotherapist, to ask that question and to be invited, for a time, into another's biography, perhaps to make a contribution to that biography. Among the most interesting aspect of your work with clients is to learn and explore other cultures. It's been said that culture is the sea we swim in. Knowing your own culture and its effects on your thinking and values is essential for the work of differentiating the values and perspectives of other cultures. Therapy offers the privilege of being invited into the wonderful diversity of human experience and to explore the answer to the question, "What is it like to be you."

The term "triangle" is a common term in family therapy and, similarly, there are three important parts to your working with a family: the nature of the family, the nature of the problem, and your nature. Who you are as an individual—your temperament and background, your experience and training, your insights and intuition—plays a significant role in how you conduct your therapy. Time and again you've heard that the therapist is the most significant agent of therapeutic change. That is certainly true in family systems therapy where the complexity and fluid interactions of all the family members require a confident therapeutic presence. Know your stuff but be yourself. Does your approach tend to be extroverted and directive or more reflective and exploratory? Therapists are individuals with their own individual styles, but what matters most is your genuine regard for your clients. Your warmth, curiosity, and encouragement, added to your training and experience, will create an environment where change, healing, and growth can happen.

Listening with Your Head, Heart, and Spirit

You listen with your *head* when you want understanding. The listening skills you've acquired in your lifetime combined with the skills and experience you are acquiring in your training will enable you to do a good job of understanding the client's story, his or her background, current circumstances, and the types of problems your client is dealing with. You have learned and practiced putting aside your preconceived ideas and perceptions about people in order to grasp the uniqueness of the person sitting in front of you. But you have also studied human behavior and the many challenges human beings share in common. Consequently, you are acquiring skill in integrating your client's unique story with the many stories that will enrich and amplify your client's understanding of his or her situation. Listening with your head helps you to better understand you clients and your clients to better understand themselves.

You listen with your *heart* when you want to connect. The limbic processes that create resonance between one individual and another enable your emotional imagination to get closer to what your client is feeling. When you allow yourself to be emotionally vulnerable to another's story, you enable your client to "feel felt," in the words of Dan Siegel. And, from *A General Theory of Love*, "If a listener quiets his neocortical chatter and allows limbic sensing to range free, melodies begin to penetrate the static of anonymity ... As the listener's resonance grows, he will catch sight of what the other sees inside that personal world, start to sense what it feels like to live there." You listen with your heart in order to connect.

You listen with your *spirit* when you want to confer value. The idea of spirit suggests our ability, as human beings, to recognize the value of other human beings. It is more than a mental or emotional grasp of the significance of the person sitting in front of you; it is a profound appreciation for the opportunity of being, for a time, present with a person on his or her journey.

James Hillman said that both the therapist and client are drawn to this therapeutic space because both experience something profoundly important there. Clearly, that may not be felt from one hour to the next, but the invitation exists to deepen one's own life so that the depth and value of another life can be more meaningfully discovered. In listening from your spirit, you open to the value of the other. Recall the teaching of Martin Buber in his book *I and Thou* (1923) that having a connection to the sacred enables one to experience another as *other* (Thou). It is in allowing oneself to be the *object* of a sentence predicated by God's creation, and not the *subject* of the sentence, that we realize our sacred kinship with humanity.

On the Sacredness of Therapy

Doctors ask, "Where does it hurt?" Historians and biographers ask, "What was it like?" Friends may ask, "How did you manage?" But few will ask, "What is it like to be you?" People don't ask that question because there's too much at stake—too much responsibility for exploring the answer. What do you do with the information? People must be paid to ask that question, and they must be trained to manage the consequences of listening, deeply listening to what it's like to be another human being. It isn't a bad thing that some people are paid to listen. Thank God for it. Asking "What is it like to be you?" carries a great deal of responsibility.

The compensation one receives from listening to a friend is in the reciprocal nature of the friendship—they will listen to you as well. The problem is that people will often protect their friends from how they truly feel. The best of friends can't be completely unguarded. We fear that our friend may catch our anxieties and depressions and may not have the stamina to fight it off or may judge us for feeling the way we do. Family members may fare better, at times, getting unguarded information. But sharing comes with a price. Family members, like friends, have a great deal at stake in the relationship. The closeness and interdependence of family members calls for caution. What price may one have to pay for getting a completely honest answer to the question, "What is it like to be you?" And if someone were genuinely willing to ask me that question, would I even want to know the answer? Do I truly want to know who I am or how I feel? There are days when the last thing I want to do is to check in with myself. It's safer just to watch television.

I suppose that what defines a professional listener or psychotherapist is the fact of being paid. But my experience is that most therapists are not primarily interested in money. That isn't why they became therapists—there are easier and more reliable ways to earn a living. I think that most therapists would also say that it isn't a simple matter of wanting to help people. Therapists in training come to terms with the reality that not everyone in therapy is helped or even genuinely wants to be helped. There is something more than money or helping people that draws certain people to the work of psychotherapy. I think it's the work itself.

What is the *work* of psychotherapy? In his book *Revisioning Psychology,* James Hillman points to the root meaning of words *psyche* as "soul" and *therapy* as "attendant" or "servant." People are drawn to the work of psychotherapy because of the significance of the work itself. In that work, one is invited to tend soul—one's own and another's. In that work, one is permitted to ask, "What is it like to be you?" Much of the education and training a therapist receives is to know how to deal with the awesome responsibility of listening to and attending to the soul of another.

The existential psychologist Erich Fromm warns therapists not to run away from the significance of their work by turning people into patients, focusing solely on symptoms, and hiding behind diagnoses and treatment plans. Fromm calls this "desacralizing." Desacralizing is robbing the soul of its depth, complexity, awe-fullness, and wonder. There are moments in therapy where it is possible to feel overwhelmed by the enormity of courage and the depths of suffering and love that exist in that place. In the presence of that sacred space I sometimes feel the urge to take off my shoes.

What is a "sacred" space? One of the meanings of the word *sacred* is to "set apart." The work of therapy requires a setting apart, not just of a particular place and time, but of a quality of openness, trust, and caring that can transform those who participate in that space. Scott Peck saw into the work of creating a sacred space when he defined love as "a willingness to extend oneself in order to facilitate one's own or another's spiritual growth." So also the authors of *A General Theory of Love* spoke to the work of creating that space when they said, "Love is not only an end for therapy; it is also the means whereby every end is reached." It is love, then—the attitude of self-extension, the "I–Thou" connection that Martin Buber described—that sets apart a particular time and place for the work of being open to truly knowing another and to the willingness to ask, "What is it like to be you?" and deeply listen to the answer.

Questions for Discussion

1. How would you begin to write an essay on what it's like to be you?
2. What gifts do you bring to this work?
3. What would help you to repair yourself from the emotional toll of doing therapy?
4. In what context have you felt valued as a unique human being?
5. What do you know for sure?
6. What values, for you, are truly important?

Becoming an Effective Multicultural Counselor

"Effective counselors understand their own cultural conditioning, the conditioning of their clients, and the sociopolitical system of which they are a part. Acquiring this understanding begins with counselors' awareness of the cultural origins of any values, biases, and attitudes they may hold. A major part of becoming a diversity-competent counselor involves challenging the idea that the values we hold are automatically true for others."[1] According to *Counseling the Culturally Diverse: Theory and Practice* (Sue & Sue, 2008), the three dimensions of competency are (1) beliefs and attitudes, (2) knowledge, and (3) skills.

Beliefs and Attitudes

- Examine and be aware of your own cultural beliefs, personal biases, and values.
- Become conscious of the tendency to transfer one's beliefs, biases, and values to others.
- Become conscious of your emotional reactions toward persons of other cultures, races, and ethnic groups.
- Seek to examine and understand the world from the vantage point of your client.
- Respect your client's religious and spiritual beliefs, customs, and values.
- Accept and value the fact of cultural diversity.
- Realize that traditional theories and techniques may not be appropriate for all clients and problems.
- Monitor your cognitive and emotional responses to culturally diverse clients throughout treatment.

Knowledge

- Learn about your client's cultural background, values, and beliefs.
- Make an effort to understand the sociopolitical and economic forces influencing your client's cultural conditioning and world views.
- Do not impose your own sociopolitical and economic biases on clients.
- Seek to understand minority family structures, hierarchies, values, and beliefs.

---

1   Corey, G. (2016). *Theory and Practice of Counseling and Psychotherapy*, p. 25.

- Seek to understand your client's community characteristics and resources.

Skills and Intervention Strategies

- Educate clients about the therapeutic process, including such things as goal setting, appropriate expectations, legal rights, and the counselor's orientation.
- Seek to use methods and strategies, and define goals that are consistent with the life experiences and cultural values of your clients.
- Modify and adapt your interventions, as needed, to accommodate cultural differences.
- Make an effort to send and receive verbal and non-verbal messages accurately.
- Seek out educational, consultative, and training experiences to enhance your knowledge and skills to work with culturally diverse client populations.

Note: In my own practice, I have found it very useful and enjoyable to understand (as much as I'm capable of understanding) my client's story and the world in which that story has taken shape and unfolds. This is certainly important in your intake process and remains an essential element of your ongoing therapy.

APPENDIX

Effective Communication
Speaking and Listening

Communication is effective when people feel heard and, ideally, valued. Thoughts, feelings, and opinions need to be understood and respected. Anything less is immature and unloving to oneself or to another. What hurts and angers us most is when our thoughts and feelings aren't acknowledged or valued. This is precisely what we communicate when we discount or disregard the feelings of others. It's tragic that effective communication can be learned easily and yet is so rare. So much needless pain and suffering could be prevented if people took the time to learn how to talk to each other.

The difficulty isn't communicating—it's communicating effectively. Emotions get in the way, and with emotions come defenses. Communicating effectively in a relationship requires helping each other to stay calm and not get defensive. This is why I keep stressing the need for practice. You may be well-qualified for a particular job, for example, but if you want to do well in your job interview, it helps to practice staying calm.

My wife and I have thought a great deal about our own communication as well as the best way to help our clients learn to communicate effectively. We've developed some very simple guidelines that work for us and for many of our clients. The guidelines are certainly not new or original to us—therapists use a variety of terms to describe the same basic skills. But we have distilled and simplified the guidelines so they are easy to remember and apply. Well, easy to remember and apply—but not without practice. You need to practice because it's hard to use a few simple behavioral guidelines to contain emotions that can be very intense and destabilizing. But it's also difficult to learn a foreign language, become a poised public speaker, or play the piano. It takes commitment and practice. People apply themselves to what they value—to what's important to them.

We can choose how we say things. We can also choose what we hear. Using the Parent, Adult, Child model is a good way to pay attention to these choices. You can address someone from the *parent* position telling them what they should do, think, or feel. You can speak from the *child* position, whining and feeling sorry for yourself. The best choice is to speak from the *adult* position, conveying *information*, not *obligation*—helping the other person to be aware of what you are feeling. Similarly, you can listen to someone from your parent, child, or adult—being judgmental, reactive, or genuinely hearing the other's feelings.

A difficult and frustrating challenge for therapists is trying to teach clients to genuinely listen to each other instead of arguing. As I mentioned previously, people get exasperated competing for whose reality gets to be reality. It's much more productive to simply state what you are feeling without trying to prove a point and to ask your listener to be open to hearing and accepting your feelings. Notice I used the word "accepting" instead of "agreeing." That is a very important distinction. We tend to get defensive when someone expresses feelings that we don't understand, hear as criticism, or disagree with. But you can't "disagree" with emotions.

Emotions simply *are*. That's one of the keys for making these communication guidelines successful—you aren't debating *perceptions*, you are simply acknowledging *feelings*. Naturally we can feel bad if we've caused someone else pain; and bad feelings can create defensiveness. People tend to want to minimize that pain by minimizing our own or the other's feelings. It's doesn't work; you'll find yourself arguing about how bad something really was, who's to blame, and who remembered the incident correctly or not. Tragically, the emotions that truly need to be expressed and heard can get lost in the debate.

The goal of a listener, therefore, is to make every effort to sidestep the need to agree or disagree with the feelings being expressed and to simply *accept* or *acknowledge* that the speaker feels a particular way. The feelings that are being discussed may seem exaggerated, irrational, or unjustified. It may be that the speaker may later wish to clarify or modify what was spoken. But the task of a good listener is not to judge but to learn, not to compete but to be curious, not to edit but to be open. And learning to become more open and vulnerable is the whole point of learning these skills.

You and your partner will practice recognizing and managing defenses. You will learn to be more trusting and less critical. And with practice, you will be able to be more vulnerable as a speaker and more open and interested as a listener. In time you'll learn to trust your skills. With a bit more time, you'll trust your partner's commitment to using those skills. Finally, it will be easier for you to trust your partner. And with increased trust, you will be amazed at how much easier it will be to step into a difficult conversation and step out again feeling better about your relationship—or if not feeling better, at least feeling heard.

Below are the guidelines. As I've said, they are simple to understand but very difficult to apply. As in learning the hand positions on the piano, a golf swing, or your computer keyboard, you could spend hours practicing and improving these skills. As I stated above, the difficulty in interpersonal communication is with your emotions. You are attempting to remember and apply some simple rules so that you're not twisted about by a tornado of feelings. Clients will spend time learning and practicing these guidelines in session to prepare them for exercises at home.

Guidelines for Effective Communication

1. Use Discretion and Good Timing

There are many levels of conversation. Casual conversations over dinner, walking and talking together, and other types of informal conversation do not require rules. "Business" talk relating to money, kids, or weekend plans does not have to conform to rigid guidelines. But when you have something very important to share, use good timing and good sense. Timing is critical. *Wait for a good time when you're most likely to have your partner's full attention.* If you're not sure if it's a good time to bring something up, ask. If you are continually put off, request (strongly, if necessary) an appointment. I recommend that couples set aside time, at least once a week, for "feeling talks." Twenty minutes might be enough time to begin with, and more time as you become comfortable with this process. It's easier to set aside the urgency of talking about troubling emotions "this minute" when you can look forward to a regularly scheduled time to share your feelings.

2. Take Turns

Too often I listen to people trying to have two conversations at once—his and hers. Remember my tennis match analogy? Slow down and take turns. Remember to breathe! *Have one speaker and one listener at a time and know which is which.* When you're the listener make sure your speaker feels heard and has finished before you take your turn. Speaker, if your listener speaks out of turn, gently redirect the focus back to you until you have finished. Be careful, however, not to talk too much at once. Keep your points clear, brief, and stay on one topic at a time. Otherwise you're "garbage-dumping," not sharing feelings. Once you feel heard, be willing to pause so that the other person can take a turn as a speaker. Learning to take turns requires practice, but there is no more important rule in communication than that each person has a chance to voice his or her emotions and concerns and feel heard and understood by the other.

The goal is for both people to "exist" in the relationship—to feel important and cared about.

3. Talk About Yourself, Your Own Feelings

Don't use *you* messages. Use *I* messages. Whenever you use the word *you*, especially in a parental or critical way, your listener is apt to become anxious and defensive. It's hard to be vulnerable. It's easy to be critical. And, for many people, it's easy to attack and blame. Don't do it! It doesn't work. The person you are attacking will be self-protective and won't listen, or he or she will attack you back. Has this ever worked for you? What's wrong with you?

Sorry for the cheesy illustration but you get the point. It *is* hard to be vulnerable, especially when you're feeling attacked. When you're engaged in a conflicted, competitive relationship, like boxers in a boxing ring, it's hard to drop your gloves.

Admittedly, being vulnerable and talking about how you feel are difficult skills to acquire. Here is my favorite phrase again—it takes lots of practice. But it's worth it for a number of reasons. Mature people appreciate vulnerability and are more apt to listen. If you are capable of honest and deep vulnerability, your listener is more likely to open his or her heart to you and to be empathic and compassionate. In other words, when you trust someone to care about you, they are more likely also. Another good reason to practice vulnerability is that it will help you to be more open to discover more about yourself.

I remember being in an angry argument years ago. My wife and I were both raising our voices, simultaneously trying to get our point across (we hadn't yet learned to use the skills I'm illustrating). We became more and more frustrated, when out of the blue I found myself tearing up. I was a younger man at the time and I hadn't been accustomed to tears. I felt ashamed and a bit surprised. I hadn't fully realized how much power I had given my wife to hurt me. I cared a great deal (perhaps too much) about her approval, and her disapproval hurt. I think that was the first time I realized that my defensive and protective anger was cushioning me from the more vulnerable pain underneath. I hadn't realized how much pain I was feeling and was surprised when it surfaced. Practicing being vulnerable paid off. I was now much more aware of my feelings.

The best book I know on depression in males has the best title I can imagine for a book on male depression. The book, by Terrence Real, is entitled *I Don't Want to Talk About It*. I could spend a great deal of time explaining why males have not been socialized to be vulnerable and why they typically have such a difficult time expressing and managing emotions, but Real has already done that. Women have had more societal permission to be vulnerable and more opportunity to practice with their girlfriends, but it isn't easy for them either. The point is that talking about emotions makes it more likely that you will feel them. Which is why most men and many women would rather avoid the process altogether.

It doesn't work. One communicates directly and responsibly or indirectly with a bad mood, angry outbursts, cold withdrawal, depression, or worse. Like most young men, my not having acquired the habit of talking about my feelings meant that most of the time I had no idea what was going on with me emotionally. Even with years of practice, it's still hard. I know that is why these guidelines appeal to me. They help me to be much less anxious about opening up. My wife has become a very skilled and empathic listener, and I'm getting better at it too. We find it's easier to have difficult conversations and are more willing, sometimes even eager, to have more. We have learned a lot about ourselves in the process and have become better friends.

Acceptance by another person helps you to accept yourself. With increased self-acceptance, you are better able to look at your real self, to see what is really there—even the things you wish weren't. Some people get confused by the idea of self-acceptance. Again, acceptance is not the same as approval. Acceptance is similar to *acknowledgment*. Self-awareness is simply acknowledging the truth about yourself. The opposite of denial, self-awareness leads to greater self-knowledge. Ideally, this knowledge opens you to psychological and spiritual growth and a greater capacity to love. So be honest. Talk about yourself, your own feelings. Be vulnerable. Describe your own emotions and experience rather than blaming others for how you feel. Other people may behave in ways that are upsetting to you, but remember, you have the choice to manage your own emotions and *respond* rather than *react*.

4. Stay in the "Here and Now"

Your feelings and opinions are important, and you have a right to be heard and to be respected. Consequently, resist the urge to "load" what you say with endless examples from the past in order to validate your feelings. *What you are feeling now is important.* When you give a history of the hurts you have suffered and the wrongs inflicted, you tend to put others on the defensive and weigh them down with guilt or fear that the past will never be forgiven or forgotten. Also be careful to stay on topic. Illustrations are dangerous. They invite debate and move the conversation away from how you are feeling in this moment. People almost always remember events differently, especially when they're in conflict. Too many conversations deteriorate into shouting matches. It's better to simply describe your emotions and try to avoid becoming entangled in a debate about what *really* happened.

Also, it's best to keep your turn short. Don't lecture. Your listener will be trying to remember what you've said in order to give you adequate feedback. Don't give your listener too much to digest or remember. Allow pauses for questions. Breathe.

And when you are done being the speaker you can say, "I'm done." More typically, I encourage clients to say, "Thanks for listening." They often resist saying that, and I understand why. People don't like overly formal or contrived-sounding sayings that they would never use at home. I get that. Figure out something better to say. The important thing is for each person to know what's going on and who's doing what. Don't be the speaker if you're supposed to be the listener. You definitely don't want two people both thinking that they are the speaker at the same time—each competing to be heard. All arguments, as far as I know, are two competing speakers, no listeners, and escalating frustration trying to be heard. The best way to turn an argument into a conversation is for someone to volunteer to be a listener. That's the missing step in conversations that dissolve into arguments. **No one is letting the other person know that they're getting it.** So the tennis match of words and feelings becomes repetitive, boring, frustrating, and infuriating until doors slam, a cold silence descends, someone uses the "D word" or collapses into tears, or the therapist is called. The reason I personally say, "Thanks for listening," is not just to let my wife know that I'm done being the speaker, although that would be reason enough. The reason I say it is because I mean it. Good listening is very hard to do. I truly value her time, effort, patience, and love, and I want her to know it.

5. Give Feedback

Let the other person know that you hear him or her, that you understand what is being said.

This doesn't mean that you have to agree with your speaker's perceptions; you simply acknowledge his or her feelings. Remember that emotions are neither right nor wrong. They simply *are*. They exist to give us information and energy. One needs to hear, respect, and try to understand them. *Should* or *should not* does not apply to feelings. You acknowledge the other's feelings by using feedback. *Feedback* is whatever you say verbally or non-verbally to convince your speaker that you're listening, interested, understanding, and caring.

Here are some suggestions for the kind of feedback that helps your speaker to feel heard and cared about. Note that the first letter of each type of feedback spells **A R C**. Think of an arc when you're listening in order to help you remember your feedback options. The letters stand for **A**ffirm, **R**epeat, or **C**larify. As the listener, giving feedback is important for two reasons: it helps you to be less defensive when you are focusing on the speaker and it helps your speaker to feel heard. You are likely to be less defensive and more open when you are listening and responding to the other's feelings instead of mentally preparing to argue back. Here are some illustrations of effective feedback:

You can **Affirm**: "I see." "Okay." "I can understand how you could feel that way."

You can **Repeat** or **Reflect**, and **Restate** what you have heard:

"You sound really angry." "You're saying that you really care about her."

"In other words, you are feeling very hurt." "Let me see if I understand you correctly ..."

You can **Clarify** or be **Curious** in order to be sure that you understand:

"I'm not sure I understand. Could you explain further?" "When, how often, have you felt this way?"

"It sounds like what you may be feeling is ..."

If you have difficulty thinking of empathic responses, below are some examples that might help. What you actually say is less important than your openness to listening with your heart and the *genuineness* of your response.

EXAMPLES OF GOOD LISTENING RESPONSES

You must feel _____.	I understand you're feeling _____.
I can understand why you could feel that way.	I can see how _____ you feel.
You sound _____.	You're telling me that you feel _____.
You look really upset.	What I hear you saying is that you feel _____.
I'm sorry you feel so _____.	I can see that _____.
You're very _____ about it.	You seem _____.
Are you feeling _____?	You must feel so _____.
You seem to need more (reassurance, comfort, attention, space, etc.) from me.	What you want is _____ (time, freedom, affection, etc.).

You can tell from these illustrations that a good listener focuses on the other person, not on themselves or the situation. Also a good listener is working to understand the other's feelings, whether they are stated and obvious or subtle and difficult to pick up. If you don't quite get what the other person is trying to describe, ask. If you think you are hearing the other person accurately, find out. Repeat back. Sometimes your speaker won't know exactly what he or she is feeling. Help out. It isn't hard. If it's an uncomfortable feeling it will boil down to what hurts and/or what's scary. Recall that anger is usually the surface symptom of the underlying emotions of hurt or fear. Let your speaker know you get it. It's even okay to interrupt, as long as it's for the purpose of clarification. You might need to say, "Could I interrupt for a moment and let you know what I'm hearing?" If your speaker is going on too long and you're having a hard time staying focused, let him know. Or gently remind the speaker that you are trying to take it all in and ask to pause for a moment so that you can give some feedback.

Okay, some of the sayings above sound like what therapists say. I understand that you don't want to feel "therapized." I also understand that when you're not used to talking to each other this way it feels strange at first. You'll get used to it. People are willing to pay for someone to really take them seriously, listen to what they have to say, and give them feedback that lets them know their feelings are important. Carl Rogers illustrated that when people feel accepted and cared about from a therapist who genuinely regards them, that whatever therapeutic approach was used, people will likely benefit from the therapy. Why not use what works, even if it feels unfamiliar and sounds therapeutic? Good relationships are therapeutic. Your careful attention to taking turns, using "I" messages, staying in the here and now, and giving good feedback will work. It has to, or things will likely blow up. Having an emotionally difficult conversation may sometimes feel like crossing a minefield. You'll make it across if you work together, go slowly and carefully, know what you're doing, allow one person to move at a time, and help each other to stay calm rather than becoming anxious or defensive.

Unfortunately, sometimes things do blow up. No matter how carefully you try to use the guidelines above, when two people feel strongly about things, painful emotions can be very difficult to manage. You're trying to work together to use a few simple rules to manage and contain some very complex, intense, and often overwhelming emotions. It isn't easy. Once again ... it takes lots of practice. So practice! I promise it will work. Don't give up. There's too much at stake not to try it.

I have worked with hundreds of couples. Some couples get the guidelines right away and begin to use them their first week of therapy. I am happy about that, but I don't usually recommend it. After the first communication lesson, I typically say with a smile, "Don't try this at home." Couples get excited about the prospect of actually being able to talk to each other successfully and are eager to try out their skills. I remember that after a few golf lessons, I was eager to get out onto the course. The unfortunate result was that I almost quit playing golf. I needed to spend more time on the driving range. I want clients to become successful in using the skills to get through a few tense conversations in the office before I encourage them to practice at home. Another metaphor might be the physician's warning not to take a cast off before the broken bone has had a chance to heal sufficiently and the patient can walk on their own strength.

From Lecture to Lab

After a few introductory "how-to" lectures, we will shift to lab work. I will ask you to talk to each other and rehearse your speaker / listener skills. At first I will be actively coaching and advising—suggesting how something might be said less offensively or heard less defensively. I may suggest topics that would be valuable to explore or feelings that need to be expressed. It's amazing and wonderful to see couples really "getting" each other, hearing feelings, responding compassionately, trusting each other, tearing up, opening up, caring, and loving. As your communication skills improve so will your trust, vulnerability, and emotional safety. When safety returns, closeness follows. It feels good to take off the boxing gloves and reach across the distance to hold each other's hand or touch each other's heart.

As skills improve, I will suggest homework, things to talk about, things to write about, conversations to try out at home, or conversations to be aware of for the next session. We will put more time between our sessions so that you have time to practice. But before that I'll want to make sure that you know what to do when things aren't working and your conversations become heated and frustrating.

6. Use "Time-Outs"

If you are being hurt or are hurting your partner, take a time-out. Go into a different room or take a walk to cool off. Time-outs are an essential tool for managing anger and keeping arguments safe. Don't use time-outs unless absolutely necessary, and always promise to give the other an appointment within 24 to 48 hours to continue the discussion, hopefully with cooler heads.

The point of saying "I need to take a time-out" is to bring your own anxiety level down so that you can continue to be effective as a speaker or listener. When an argument becomes overheated it is difficult to hold on to one's "adult." Many people abort a painful argument by leaving with harsh words and slamming doors. Others raise voices, call names, threaten, or worse. Don't let it get that far. As soon as you become conscious of the tension in your body that signals your anger or anxiety level rising out of control, take a time-out. Use the words, "I need to take a time-out."

When people leave an argument in anger or hostility, it typically creates acute separation anxiety for the other. Rational people are reduced to acting like children, blocking doorways, hiding car keys, hurling insults, or becoming violent. These episodes can cause physical or emotional injury and result in people calling the police or an attorney. Again, don't let it get that far. Saying, "I'm taking a time-out" is a promise to continue the conversation at a later time after you've calmed down. It's much less stressful for your partner to hear that promise than a door slamming. It tells your partner that you're not going anywhere, they are not being abandoned or punished, the conversation isn't being avoided or permanently postponed; you simply need time to bring your anxiety level down. Don't fool yourself. You are not ready to resume a difficult conversation for at least 20 minutes. More time is better. If it's late at night, you shouldn't even have begun. I promise that as you get used to having more successful conversations you'll become more confident that you can table a conversation and resume it at a better time. Work together; help each other to stay calm. As both of you are reassured that you will successfully conclude the conversation when you're calm, time-outs become much easier.

7. Have a "Postmortem"

I can appreciate the fact that the term "postmortem" is not normally associated with couple communication (unless, perhaps, the communication gets way out of hand). The term is normally used in the medical profession to determine the cause of a death. I am using the term here to suggest that when communication has "died" for some reason, it would be good to find out why.

A "postmortem" is one of the most important learning and healing tools in a relationship. If an underlying reason for the outbreak of conflict is un-accessed or unexpressed emotions, a postmortem is the process of discussing and exploring those emotions once they have surfaced. It's a time, from shortly after an argument to a day or two later, when you sit down with your partner to talk about why the argument happened, what you were really arguing about, and what you can learn from it. Arguments often happen spontaneously and unexpectedly because important information or emotions have been avoided and need to be discussed. Conflict helps to bring that information to the surface. *Your commitment to dealing with the information brought to light in conflict will make the difference between a boring, stagnant relationship and a healthy, growing one.*

After a spat, it's normal to want to forget the angry words and hurt feelings. Couples avoid talking about their feelings afterwards for fear that the argument will start up again. In some cases a spat isn't very complicated, mostly just embarrassing, and there isn't much to gain by discussing it. When the argument is heated, however, and harsh words are said, it's a mistake to ignore it and hope that things will just get better. They usually won't. Very likely those unresolved feelings will resurface. A postmortem is an attempt to talk about these feelings safely with a view to understanding deeper levels of the conflict. Ideally, a good postmortem will not only help to resolve conflict but also create a context where healing can occur. The goal of a postmortem is to be more aware of emotional triggers—to learn more about yourself and the other. A postmortem will also help you to

1. discover you and your partner's deeper feelings, needs, and wounds;
2. acknowledge your part in the conflict, apologize if need be, and determine what you might have done differently or will do differently in the future;
3. create greater trust and closeness;
4. open the door to resolving specific issues; and
5. reaffirm your commitment to working and growing together.

Preparing for the Postmortem

Through writing, reflecting, praying, etc., take time to consider your deeper feelings, issues, ongoing themes, and needs. Realize that you cannot ask someone to take responsibility to meet all of your needs, but you can ask that person to hear and accept your feelings. In "transactional analysis" language, this is talking from your "adult" as opposed to your scolding, controlling "parent" or your needy, whining "child." You may want to admit to having "lost your adult" during the argument when you attacked the other person or stormed out of the room. You will want to try again to listen to your partner's feelings, this time from a more contained "adult" position.

In an environment of safety and openness, you will find yourselves being more open to hearing deeper patterns and themes in your dialogue. This type of listening can be very therapeutic. With increased trust and vulnerability, you are more likely to recall and feel the pain of old injuries from childhood. You cannot help being affected by wounds from the past. I've already listed many of the reasons this occurs. Becoming conscious of these old wounds, discussing them, and feeling the feelings, however unpleasant, is how therapy works. In the same way, a good marriage can not only be exceptionally close and satisfying, it can also be very healing.

You can learn a great deal from a good postmortem. An even richer reward than clearing the air, sharing your feelings, and being reassured that you have been heard, is the wonderful sense of renewed trust, closeness, and affection between you. A good postmortem results in a deeper understanding of the underlying themes that keep coming up in your relationship so that you can make more loving decisions in the future. Remember the lesson about reenactment discussed previously? Healing happens when you recognize those trigger issues, identify where you're sensitive, and ask your partner to be more aware and considerate. As both of you work to be more aware of the other and practice making more sensitive and loving decisions, your relationship will become the most vital and joyful experience of your life, and the two of you will find, in the quality of each other's friendship, a resource for healing and well-being that is astounding.

In your postmortem you will do some emotional archeology. Conflict usually exists in layers. What you find yourself arguing about on the surface, especially if the conflict is intense, is usually charged with emotional content from deeper down. Below are the typical strata or layers in the archeology of a relationship. Don't be surprised if the vulnerability and trust you have been working to acquire create a context in which you will gain some amazing insights and reach even deeper levels of trust, intimacy, and healing. The reason we focus on process in therapy is to give you the skills you need to safely and successfully dig deeper into the layers of your relationship and unearth the important emotions, themes, and wounds that may be buried there.

The Archeology of Relationship

Conversations can become very difficult if a *problem* being discussed is the most recent illustration of an underlying and ongoing *theme*. In this sense, the problem is simply the surface of layered experience and emotion. It's useful, at times, to think archeologically about the deeper layers beneath. Here's a guide to your excavation.

Problems: The surface issues and challenges of negotiating how best to manage time, money, roles and responsibilities, kids, in-laws, your sexual relationship, and so forth. Frequently couples report that the problems in their relationship revolve around differences in how to manage their time, raise their children, negotiate finances, etc. Sometimes this is actually true. If a couple is losing their home or they have a very sick child, this is certainly the most pressing problem. Most of the time, however, the problem in the relationship isn't at the "problem level" it's with the "process"—that is, how successfully the couple communicate about the problem.

Process: How well the two of you are able to discuss and negotiate issues. Are you able to manage your psychological defenses—keep your critical "parent" or hurt "child" out of the conversation and stay in your "adult"?

Pain: This is a layer of painful and difficult emotions that persist from one argument to another and often underlie chronic conflict and recurring relationship themes. It isn't that my spouse forgot to do something that is important to me—it's that he or she forgot *again* or keeps forgetting. It is these ongoing and relentless hurts and irritations that become relationship themes. When a small offense becomes the most recent example of a continuing pattern, it's easy to lose faith in the other, to feel less important and less loved. When a problem surfaces at the problem level, it may become the most recent illustration of an ongoing theme.

Past: The emotional wounds from childhood and past relationships that overlay and intensify the pain of your recurring relationship themes. This layer also includes the effects of your childhood conditioning and early attachments. The emotional and relational patterns that we internalize as children continue to exert an influence on how we experience and respond to our present relationships. Understanding our past emotional learning is very important in recognizing how our present emotional reactions may be triggered and intensified from the past.

Personalities: The differences in your innate temperaments with corresponding differences in your goals, values, ways of managing stress, and ways of loving. *Who* you are determines *how* you are—or at least how you can be. Our inherited temperament inclines us toward certain styles of relating and informs our values, our appetites for certain activities, and, most importantly, the diverse ways that we express and experience love.

Guidelines for Good Communication Handout

On the next page I've included a one-page handout on Guidelines for Good Communication. You're welcome to copy the guidelines for your own use and give it to your clients. Many clients are reluctant to do much reading, so I've discovered that giving them a condensed version of the guidelines seems to work well. I jokingly comment that "this is the textbook for the course." I go on to say that after a brief lecture on communication skills and emotions, we'll get down to the "lab work" of facing each other and practicing the skills. The sooner a couple is able to progress having safe, successful conversations, the sooner they won't need you. Remember that your ultimate goal with your couple client is to become redundant.

Guidelines for Good Communication Handout

I've condensed the most important steps to good communication to these seven guidelines. The goal is to reduce defensiveness by taking turns and practicing openness in both speaking and listening.

SPEAKER	LISTENER
1. Use good timing and discretion	4. Give feedback
2. Talk about yourself (your own feelings)	5. Wait your turn to be speaker
3. Stay current, be brief	
Goal: to be vulnerable, to be open, to truly trust your feelings and concerns are being heard and accepted	**Goal:** to hear what your speaker is saying, to truly hear what your speaker is saying, and to enable your speaker to feel heard
Briefly state the context i.e., When you ... When this happens ... Sometimes I feel ...	**Listen with your heart** Try to validate, comfort, and reassure, or at least try to be curious, not competitive
Identify your feelings i.e., I feel angry, scared, hurt, happy	**Give feedback** Feedback is about what you hear, not what you think. Think about creating an **A.R.C.** between you and the speaker **A A**ffirm or **A**cknowledge **R R**epeat back or reflect **C C**larify, be **C**urious

Taking Turns

Making the transition from one speaker to another can be tricky. It feels unfamiliar and a little too formal to take turns, but it is very important to know who is doing what. You are trying to help each other to remember the rules, not to get competitive, and to remember that *when you're the listener, you're not the speaker.*

The best way to do this, if you are the speaker, is to say, "Thanks for listening," or "I'm done," or something similar that lets the listener know that he or she can take a turn. If you are the listener, politely ask if your speaker feels heard and if you can take your turn being the speaker.

DON'TS FOR THE SPEAKER	DON'TS FOR THE LISTENER
Tax the listener with too much info	Square the record, justify, defend
Use examples and illustrations	Grab the speaker role
Hog the speaker role	Resist letting information in
Use the speaker role as an opportunity to berate the listener	Be technically correct with no heart
Go on and on without pausing	Require agreement
	Have agendas in listening responses

6. **Take a time-out** when things get too frustrating and you need time to cool down (not less than 20 minutes or more than 48 hours or some other agreed-upon time).
7. **Have a postmortem** after your time-out or later in the week to discuss how you felt during the argument, to reassure each other that you are committed to listening and working things out, and to discuss what you have learned about yourself or the other during the argument.

Discussion Questions About Emotions

1. Of the primary emotions—anger, fear, and sadness—what emotions are you most likely to be conscious of during conflict?
2. How do you normally express these emotions?
3. How do others typically react when you express these emotions?
4. At some point do you become aware of any underlying emotions or ongoing emotional themes? What emotions or themes are you aware of?
5. As you were growing up, what messages did you receive from your parents about anger? About fear? About sadness?
6. How do these parental messages affect your ability to recognize and express emotions now?
7. What emotions expressed by others are most difficult for you to listen to and what reaction do they trigger in you?

Discussion Questions About Defenses

1. What type of psychological defense do you find yourself using most often?
2. What other defenses have you used?

3. What percent of the time are you able to manage your defenses?
4. What defense do you most dislike in others?
5. What helps you to become aware that you are being defensive?
6. When you are conscious of being defensive, are you able to admit it? Are you able to manage your defensives?
7. What techniques could you try in order to work on becoming less defensive?

Discussion Questions About Messages

1. What are some of the unspoken messages that are most likely to upset you?
2. When you are upset, what indirect messages are you likely to express?
3. How often do you find yourself saying something you didn't intend to say?
4. In your significant relationships, how often do these mixed messages cause conflicts?
5. How much time do you spend attempting to resolve these conflicts?
6. What messages are difficult for you to express?
7. What three changes would make a big improvement in your relationship?

Common "Feeling Words"

ANGER	SADNESS	FEAR
GRUMPY	LOW	HESITANT
Annoyed	Moody	Insecure
Irritated	Discouraged	Suspicious
Cross	Disappointed	Worried
Provoked	Somber	Nervous
Offended	Sullen	Threatened
Indignant	Dreary	Alarmed
Angry	Melancholy	Apprehensive
Frustrated	Hurt	Anxious
Bitter	Hopeless	Hysterical
Mad	Heavy-hearted	Fearful
Enraged	Sad	Scared
Infuriated	Depressed	Frightened
Outraged	Despairing	Panicky
PASSION	**SERENITY**	**CONFIDENCE**
Close	Relaxed	Encouraged
Tender	Calm	Reassured
Warm	Serene	Trusting

Affectionate	Comfortable	Hopeful
Loving	Peaceful	Secure
Seductive	Contented	Confident
Aroused	Restful	Bold
Passionate	Well-being	Courageous
Excited	Accepting	Carefree
Inspired	Settled	Optimistic
Exhilarated	Relieved	Enthusiastic
Ecstatic	Satisfied	Energized

Modified Differentiation of Self Scale*

These are questions concerning your thoughts and feelings about yourself and relationships with others. Please read each statement carefully and decide how much the statement is *generally true* of you on a 1 (*not at all*) to 6 (*very true*) scale. If you believe that an item does not pertain to you (e.g., you are not currently married or in a committed relationship, or one or both of your parents are deceased), please answer the item according to your best guess about what your thoughts and feelings would be in that situation. Be sure to answer every item and try to be as honest and accurate as possible in your responses.

1. People have remarked that I'm overly emotional.   1 2 3 4 5 6
2. I have difficulty expressing my feelings to people I care for.   1 2 3 4 5 6
3. I often feel inhibited around my family.   1 2 3 4 5 6
4. I tend to remain pretty calm even under stress.   1 2 3 4 5 6
5. I'm likely to smooth over or settle conflicts between two people whom I care about.   1 2 3 4 5 6
6. When someone close to me disappoints me, I withdraw from him or her for a time.   1 2 3 4 5 6
7. No matter what happens in my life, I know that I'll never lose my sense of who I am.   1 2 3 4 5 6
8. I tend to distance myself when people get too close to me.   1 2 3 4 5 6
9. It has been said (or could be said) of me that I am still very attached to my parent(s).   1 2 3 4 5 6
10. I wish that I weren't so emotional.   1 2 3 4 5 6
11. I usually do not change my behavior simply to please another person.   1 2 3 4 5 6
12. My spouse or partner could not tolerate it if I were to express my true feelings.   1 2 3 4 5 6
13. Whenever there is a problem in my relationship, I'm anxious to get it settled right away.   1 2 3 4 5 6
14. At times my feelings get the best of me and I have trouble thinking clearly.   1 2 3 4 5 6

15. In an argument, I can separate my thoughts about the issue from my feelings about the person.   1 2 3 4 5 6

16. I'm often uncomfortable when people get too close to me.   1 2 3 4 5 6

17. It's important for me to keep in touch with my parents regularly.   1 2 3 4 5 6

18. At times, I feel as if I'm riding an emotional roller coaster.   1 2 3 4 5 6

19. There's no point in getting upset about things I cannot change.   1 2 3 4 5 6

20. I'm concerned about losing my independence in intimate relationships.   1 2 3 4 5 6

21. I'm overly sensitive to criticism.   1 2 3 4 5 6

22. When my spouse or partner is away for too long, I feel like I am missing a part of me.   1 2 3 4 5 6

23. I'm fairly self-accepting.   1 2 3 4 5 6

24. I often feel that my spouse or partner wants too much from me.   1 2 3 4 5 6

25. I try to live up to my parents' expectations.   1 2 3 4 5 6

26. If I have had an argument with my spouse or partner, I tend to think about it all day.   1 2 3 4 5 6

27. I am able to say no to others even when I feel pressured by them.   1 2 3 4 5 6

28. When one of my relationships becomes very intense, I feel the urge to run away from it.   1 2 3 4 5 6

29. Arguments with my parent(s) or sibling(s) can still make me feel awful.   1 2 3 4 5 6

30. If someone is upset with me, I can't seem to let it go easily.   1 2 3 4 5 6

31. I'm less concerned that others approve of me than I am about doing what I think is right.   1 2 3 4 5 6

32. I would never consider turning to any of my family members for emotional support.   1 2 3 4 5 6

33. I find myself thinking a lot about my relationship with my spouse or partner.   1 2 3 4 5 6

34. I'm very sensitive to being hurt by others.   1 2 3 4 5 6

35. My self-esteem really depends on how others think of me.   1 2 3 4 5 6

36. When I'm with my spouse or partner, I often feel smothered.   1 2 3 4 5 6

37. I worry about people close to me getting sick, hurt, or upset.   1 2 3 4 5 6

38. I often wonder about the kind of impression I create.   1 2 3 4 5 6

39. When things go wrong, talking about them usually makes it worse.   1 2 3 4 5 6

40. I feel things more intensely than others do. | 1 | 2 | 3 | 4 | 5 | 6 |
41. I usually do what I believe is right regardless of what others say. | 1 | 2 | 3 | 4 | 5 | 6 |
42. Our relationship might be better if my spouse or partner would give me the space I need. | 1 | 2 | 3 | 4 | 5 | 6 |
43. I tend to feel pretty stable under stress. | 1 | 2 | 3 | 4 | 5 | 6 |

Differentiation of Self Inventory Subscale Composition
(underlined means reverse scored): Emotional Reactivity:
1, 6, 10, 14, 18, 21, 26, 30, 34, 38, 40
I Position: 4, 7, 11, 15, 19, 23, 27, 31, 35, 41, 43
Emotional Cutoff: 2, 3, 8, 12, 16, 20, 24, 28, 32, 36, 39, 42
Fusion with Others: 5, 9, 13, 17, 22, 25, 29, 33, 37

By permission of the authors: E. Skowron and M. Friedlander, February 16, 1998.

Parenting Plan

A parenting plan is a good way to help your children learn positive and negative consequences for behavior and be responsible for their choices with a token "economy." Below are ideas for setting up and maintaining a parenting plan.

Please list the behaviors you want your child to stop doing. Here are some typical categories of behavior:

Dawdling
1.
2.
3.

Disrespect
1.
2.
3.

Disobedience
1.
2.
3.

Deception
1.
2.
3.

Other
1.
2.

Please rewrite the above behaviors in positive terms as behaviors you want to see.
1.
2.
3.
4.
5.
6.
7.
8.

What positive consequences would you like to give your child for meeting behavioral goals?
1.
2.
3.
4.
5.
6.

What negative consequences will you apply for not meeting expectations? Consider escalating consequences for non-compliance.
1.
2.
3.
4.
5.
6.

If you are a two-parent family, how will you decide how the consequences will be administered?

_____
_____
_____
_____
_____
_____

If you are a two-parent family, how will you "huddle" when you disagree on behaviors and consequences?

_____
_____
_____
_____
_____
_____

How will you determine whether your parenting plan is working, staying current, or needs modification?

_____

_____

_____

_____

_____

_____

Marriage Survey

Instructions

The checklist below is designed to give you and your spouse the opportunity to evaluate aspects of your relationship that you would like to improve. There is a checklist for each of you.

1. First, please go through your own checklist and place a checkmark next to those areas that you would like your spouse to pay closer attention to.
2. Next, go back over the list and place an X next to items you believe your spouse has checked.
3. You may decide to switch checklists to see what areas your spouse is checking as well as how well you communicate with each other (if the checkmarks on one list match the Xs on the other). Or, you may prefer to hold on to the checklists and share them with each other in therapy.

Marital Survey

Check only the things lacking in your relationship but that you WISH your relationship had.

I. Daily Meaningful Conversation
_____ tell me how s/he feels in more depth
_____ really talk to me at least once a day for 15 minutes
_____ talk to me alone each day (just the two of us, no TV, no kids present)
_____ tell me when s/he is hurt or depressed
_____ tell me good things as well as complaints
_____ not complain so much
_____ not argue with everything I say
_____ not always have to have the last word
_____ listen more and talk less
_____ talk more about ideas, current events, etc., rather than on routine problems
_____ talk more about spiritual things to me
_____ let me have at least a half hour of solitude each day
_____ not talk to me about problems for the first 15 minutes we are together in the evening

Adapted from Shepherd's House Counseling Center, "Marital Survey."

____ tell me that s/he loves me more often
____ compliment me and "notice" me more often
____ indicate more often that s/he really understands what I'm saying
____ care more about my problems and concerns
____ not take me for granted so much

_____
_____
_____

II. Constructive Conflict
____ not always avoid a confrontation with me
____ not always get mad when we disagree
____ not always insist on winning
____ not pout so much
____ not shout at me
____ not leave the house as a way of winning
____ not throw up my past mistakes at me during an argument
____ try to understand my way of seeing things about which we disagree
____ listen more and talk less
____ not threaten me during an argument (i.e., with leaving, divorce, etc.)
____ let me win sometimes
____ be able to disagree and let it go at that
____ not attack me personally (i.e., calling me names, etc.)
____ not stock up issues and argue about several things at once
____ not start crying as a way of winning
____ not act like a martyr
____ not use guilt-producing statements like "if it weren't for you, I would be happy"
____ not always hide his/her negative, hurt, angry feelings and pretend to be happy
____ not hold things in and finally explode once in awhile
____ not hold things in and show anger in mean but subtle little ways

III. Sexual Intercourse
____ be able to talk to me about our sexual life without getting too defensive
____ share his/her real feelings about our sexual relationship
____ tell me more about his/her likes and dislikes in terms of sexual behaviors
____ be more clear about how s/he likes to be turned on during foreplay
____ be willing to be more experimental in our sexual behavior with each other
____ listen more when I tell him/her what I like and don't like
____ spend more time in warming up or foreplay before intercourse
____ be more sensitive to my readiness for intercourse
____ not be in such a hurry
____ not take so long to warm up
____ have intercourse with me more often
____ have intercourse with me less often
____ initiate sexual play more often, be more aggressive
____ be more passive, sometimes let me initiate sexual play
____ be more seductive earlier in the evening
____ not make excuses to avoid sexual intimacy (i.e., headaches, tiredness, etc.)

_____
_____
_____

IV. Nonsexual Touching

_____ kiss me goodbye in the morning

_____ kiss me hello in the evening

_____ not always expect sexual play whenever we embrace or kiss

_____ show me more physical attention without expecting to progress to intercourse

_____ not display so much physical attention in public

_____ display more affection in public

_____ sit with me more in the evening

_____

_____

_____

V. Entertainment

_____ be willing to go out more often

_____ be willing to take more vacations

_____ be more willing to do things I like to do

_____ be more sociable

_____ go off with me for a weekend alone more often

_____ be willing to stay home more often

_____ spend less time doing his/her own things (i.e., golf without me)

_____ let me feel free to do my own things more often and not make me feel guilty about it

_____ not be such a loud mouth or so obnoxious; be more sensitive in public

_____

_____

_____

VI. Spiritual Life

_____ be more interested in spiritual things

_____ pray with me more often

_____ read the scriptures and have devotions with me more often

_____ initiate devotions and not wait for me to do it

_____ become more involved in spiritual activities

_____ become less involved in spiritual activities

_____ not nag me so much about changing some things in my life

_____ be less critical of me spiritually

_____ share more of his/her spiritual thoughts and feelings with me

_____ be more open and less superficial when we pray together

_____ be more willing to confess sins and weaknesses

_____ be more open with acquaintances who don't share our faith

_____ not act so pious with our friends

_____ be less hypocritical

_____ participate more with me in my faith

_____ be more humble, less arrogant

_____ be less defensive when I point out areas in which he/she needs to grow

_____

_____

_____

VII. Finances

_____ be more thrifty

_____ not be so tight about money

_____ give me more say-so in financial decisions

_____ take over more of the financial decision-making

_____ not use the credit card so much

_____ establish more charge accounts

_____ not get so angry about unexpected bills

_____ not gamble so much in business ventures, stocks, etc.

_____ take a job or contribute more to family income

_____ work less and spend more time with the family

_____ agree that we can each have a little money each week that we don't have to account for and can spend on anything we want

_____ sit down and set financial goals with me; make a budget

_____ agree to buy or spend more money on _____

_____

_____

_____

VIII. Children

_____ agree to have a child or more children soon

_____ not insist on having a child or more children and quit bugging me about it

_____ agree to use a different birth control method

_____ be more strict in disciplining the children

_____ be less strict in disciplining the children

_____ spend more time with the children

_____ talk more to the children about their interests and problems

_____ not yell at the children so much

_____ show more physical affection to the children

_____ be more understanding of the children

_____ use another method to discipline the children

_____ not show favoritism to one child

_____

_____

_____

IX. Personal Appearance

_____ lose weight

_____ dress more neatly

_____ shave, bathe, etc., more frequently

_____ look more attractive in the evening

_____ use more deodorant or perfume

_____

_____

_____

X. In-Laws

_____ not spend so much time with his/her parents

_____ be less dependent on his/her parents

_____ not insist on attending so many family functions

_____ be more willing to move farther away from his/her parents

_____ not compare me with his/her parents

_____

_____

_____

XI. Dealing with Problems

_____ not concentrate so much on problems; talk more about our strengths

_____ admit that we have serious problems in our marriage

_____ agree to seek professional help for our individual or marital problems

_____

_____

_____

XII. Use this space to bring up any other topics not addressed above.

_____

_____

_____

_____

_____

_____

_____

_____

_____

_____

_____

_____

_____

_____

_____

_____

INDEX

A

ABCDE model, 20
"actualization tendency", 8
Adler, Alfred, 8, 12, 109
Amini, F., 6, 23, 76, 77, 84, 99
angst, 46–47
attachment, 23–25
  styles, 25–27
Attachment (Bowlby), 9
attraction, 23–25

B

"The Basic I.D.", 19
"behavioral" stories, 2
behavior-oriented therapies, 90
belonging
  healthy marriages, 75–77
Berne, Eric, 60–63
The Body Never Lies (Miller), 91
The Body Remembers (Rothschild), 91
Bowen, Murray, 12, 109, 116
Bowlby, John, 9–10
brain
  and complex memories, 11
  as story teller, 3
Briggs-Myers, Isabel, 29
Briggs-Myers, Katharine, 29
Buber, Martin, 120
Burns, David, 89

C

Campbell, Joseph, 11
catharsis, 16
causal idea, 7
choices, 32–33
Christensen, Andrew, 72, 87, 94–95, 101
circular causality, 67

cognitive-behavioral family therapy, 110
"cognitive" stories, 2
communication
  confusing messages, 55–57
  psychological defenses, 58–60
  transactional analysis, 60–63
conflict
  -free relationship, 82
  purpose of, 81–85
content and process, in relationships, 67–71
counseling session, relationships, 65–66
The Courage to Create (May), 10–11
Covey, Steven, 8
Cozolino, Louis, 3, 15–16, 46

D

Damasio, Antonio, 81, 83, 91
deals
  feelings and, 79
  fun and, 79
  healthy marriages, 79
  making, 79–80
defenses, psychological, 58–60
The Denial of Death (Becker), 11
The Developing Mind: How relationships and the brain interact to shape who we are (Siegel), 9, 46, 105
Dickens, Charles, 12
differentiation
  described, 12
  external, 12
  internal, 12
Do I Have to Give Up Me to Be Loved by You?, 70

E

The Eighth Habit: From Effectiveness to Greatness (Covey), 8
Ellis, Albert, 20
emotional honesty, 49–53
emotionally focused therapy, 90–91
emotional memory, 31–32
emotions
  color of, 39–43
  primary, 37–39
  secondary, 43–46
Enhancing Couples (Christensen), 87–90
enjoying, healthy marriages, 77
Erikson, Erik, 8
Escape from Freedom (Fromm), 10
evidence-based approach, 8
experiential family therapy, 109
external differentiation, 12

F

families
  defined, 106
  differentiation, 108, 116–117
  finding the best approach to treating client's, 113–116
  genogram, 118
  motivation, and openness to change, 108
family dynamics, 106–107
family rituals, 117–118
family roles, 117
family rules, 117
family stressors, 107
family systems, 107–108

family therapy
  eight approaches, 109–111
  integrative approach,
    110–111
Feeling Good (Burns), 89
fight and flight defenses,
  58–59
Frankl, Victor, 18
Freud, Sigmund, 77–78
Fromm, Erich, 10, 18

G

Games People Play (Berne),
  60
A General Theory of Love
  (Lewis, Amini and
  Lannon), 5, 23, 24, 26,
  76, 77, 81, 84, 99, 120,
  121
genogram, 118
Getting the Love You Want
  (Hendrix), 10, 89
Gottman, John, 71–72, 79
Gray, John, 53
Great Expectations
  (Dickens), 12
"guiding fiction,", 8

H

healing (psychotherapy),
  15–17
healthy marriages
  belonging, 76–77
  deals, feelings, and fun,
    79
  described, 75–76
  enjoying, 77
  making deals, 79–80
  practicing playfulness,
    77–79
  valuing, 76
helping couples
  applying Christensen's
    strategies, 98–104
  approaches to therapy, 88
  behavior-oriented
    therapies, 90
  emotionally focused
    therapy, 90–91
  insight-oriented
    therapies, 89–90
  principles of change,
    93–95
  strategies, 97–98

thoughts, feelings,
  behaviors, 89
where do we start?—
  where are we headed),
  91–93
your next session, 96–97
your treatment plan,
  87–88
helping (psychotherapy),
  19–21
Hendrix, Harville, 10,
  89–90
Hero with a Thousand
  Faces (Campbell), 11
Hillman, James, 11, 121
Hillman, Jim, 8
His Way—Her Way, 80
holding (psychotherapy),
  17–19
Horney, Karen, 12
human development
  and causal idea, 7
  and teleological story,
    7–8
human potential movement,
  5

I

I and Thou (Buber), 120
individuation, 8
insight-oriented therapies,
  89–90
internal differentiation, 12

J

Jung, Carl, 8, 11

K

Kierkegaard, Soren, 10, 18
Klein, Melanie, 10
Kottler, Jeff, 18

L

language
  psychological, 4, 5
  and stories, 2
Lannon, R., 76, 77, 84, 99
Lazarus, Arnold, 19–20
Lewis, T., 76, 77, 84, 99
Looking for Spinoza
  (Damasio), 81, 83,
  91
Loss (Bowlby), 9

M

Maslow, Abraham, 5, 8
May, Rollo, 11, 17, 18
McAdams, Dan, 9–10, 11
McKee, Robert, 9
memory, 31–32. see also
  brain
messages, confusing, 55–57
Miller, Alice, 91
motive, 34–35
Myers–Briggs Type Indicator
  (MBTI), 29–30

N

narrative family therapy, 109
neural integration, 16
The Neuroscience of
  Psychotherapy
  (Cozolino), 3, 46

O

On Being a Therapist
  (Kottler), 18

P

Parent, Adult, Child model,
  60–63
Peck, Scott, 13, 50, 99, 108
perceptions, negotiating,
  33–34
personalities, relationships,
  72
playfulness, 77–79
primary emotions, 37–39
psychodynamic and
  transgenerational
  family therapy, 109
"psychodynamic" stories,
  2, 4
psychological defenses,
  58–60
psychological languages, 4, 5
psychology
  existential, 47
  language of, 9
  overview, 8–9
The Psychology of Love
  (Sternberg), 75, 76
psychotherapy
  healing, 15–17
  helping, 19–21
The Purpose Driven Life
  (Warren), 8

R

Rank, Otto, 18
reenactment, 30–31
relationships
  conflict-free, 82
  content and process,
    67–72
  counseling session, 65–66
  personalities, 72
  problems, 72–73
  "relaxation training,",
    71
Revisioning Psychology
  (Hillman), 121
The Road Less Traveled
  (Peck), 13, 50, 99, 108
Rogers, Carl, 5, 6, 68, 92
  "actualization tendency,",
    8
  person-centered
    approach, 17
Rothschild, Babette, 91

S

Satir, Virginia, 109
schema, 1

secondary emotions, 43–46
"Self,", 8
self-actualization, 8, 12–13
Separation (Bowlby), 9
The Seven Principles for
  Making Marriage Work
  (Gottman), 71–72,
  75, 79
"sharing intimacies,", 76
Siegel, Dan, 1, 9, 46, 105, 120
solution-focused family
  therapy, 110
The Soul's Code (Hillman),
  8, 11
splitting, 10
Star Wars, 11
Sternberg, R., 75–76
  The Stories We Live By
    (McAdams), 9–10, 11
Story (McKee), 9
strategic family therapy, 110
structural family therapy,
  109–110

T

talk therapy, 3
  and healing, 16

Tannen, Deborah, 53
teleological story, 7–8
temperament, 29–30
therapy. *see also*
    psychotherapy
  as talking cure, 3
  listening with head,
    heart, and spirit, 120
  sacredness of, 120–121
  stories in, 3
  transactional analysis,
    60–63
truth, 34–35

V

valuing, healthy marriages,
  76
vulnerability, 32

W

Warren, Rick, 8
Whitaker, Carl, 109
Winnicott, Donald, 17

www.ingramcontent.com/pod-product-compliance
Lightning Source LLC
Chambersburg PA
CBHW081108220326
41598CB00038B/7273